The
Autism
Puzzle

The Autism Puzzle

CONNECTING THE DOTS BETWEEN
ENVIRONMENTAL TOXINS AND
RISING AUTISM RATES

BRITA BELLI

SEVEN STORIES PRESS
New York

A Seven Stories Press First Edition

Seven Stories Press
140 Watts Street
New York, NY 10013
www.sevenstories.com

College professors may order examination copies of Seven Stories Press titles for a free six-month trial period. To order, visit www.sevenstories.com/ textbook or send a fax on school letterhead to (212) 226-1411.

Book design by Elizabeth DeLong

Library of Congress Cataloging-in-Publication Data
Belli, Brita.
The autism puzzle : connecting the dots between environmental toxins and rising autism rates / Brita Belli. -- 1st ed.
    p. ; cm.
Includes bibliographical references and index.
ISBN 978-1-60980-391-9 (hardback)
I. Title.
[DNLM: 1. Autistic Disorder--etiology. 2. Environmental Pollutants-- adverse effects. WS 350.8.P4]
LC classification not assigned
616.85'882--dc23
                                    2011044260

Printed in the United States

9 8 7 6 5 4 3 2 1

In loving memory of my father, Howard Jon Brundage

CONTENTS

❖

The Missing Percentage
Why Genetics Alone Can't Explain the Steady Climb

In Lewis Carroll's *Alice's Adventures in Wonderland*, the lovable Hatter (Carroll didn't actually call his character the "Mad Hatter," though most people do) was based on eighteenth century hatmakers. Hatters were "mad" for a reason: they toiled in poorly ventilated rooms using orange-colored mercury nitrate to cure fur into felt, which could be more easily shaped and manipulated into the latest fashions. The process was called "carroting" due to the solution's color. After years spent shaping hats, these workers began exhibiting signs of neurological damage—stumbling, slurred speech, and shaking that became known in the city of Danbury, Connecticut, once the hat-making capital of the world, as "the Danbury shakes." In its heyday, the city produced five million hats per year. When the hat factories closed, the shaky legacy remained. Mercury from the factories' wastewater settled in the sediment of the city's Still River. "You could tell the color of the hats you were making by looking at the Still River," eighty-six-year-old Bob Reynolds, a former hat factory worker, told local newspaper *The News-*

Times. Ted Hammer whose uncle counted several hatters among his friends recalled how the men would share a drink in the factory's back room, some shaking so badly they could hardly hold their glasses of whiskey: "My uncle used to tell me [in regards to his shaking friend], 'Hold his glass. Don't let whiskey go to waste.'" A few drinks in, the shakes improved, but they never went away.[1]

A host of symptoms follow within hours of inhaling mercury vapors, including tremors, corrosive bronchitis with fever chills, abdominal cramping with diarrhea, and central nervous system damage that can lead to visual and psychotic disturbances. Women who become pregnant by men who are chronically exposed to mercury vapors have higher rates of spontaneous abortion.[2]

Direct exposure to mercury in the workplace is far less prevalent now than it was in the day of the Danbury hatters. Mercury poisoning can still occur in factories that produce chlorine, medical equipment, fluorescent lights, pesticides, dental amalgams, and certain chemicals, but stories like that of the hatters have led to safety regulations meant to lower employees' risk.[3] However, the general population is increasingly subject to subtler, yet equally damaging, chemical hazards present in our food and environment: mercury in the fish we eat and bisphenolA (BPA) in our canned food; phthalates and flame retardants we breathe in our household dust; water-based disinfectants we inhale while showering and insecticides we inadvertently absorb while treating our homes and pets. Doctors and scientists have begun to identify a relationship between increased exposures to such chemicals with simultaneous increases in various illnesses and disorders in children—in particular, autism.

Autism affects an average of 1 in 110 kids in the US according to the most recent 2006 data from the Centers for Disease Control and Prevention[4] with similar numbers in Europe, Asia, and the rest of North America[5]—a 57 percent increase since 2002.[6] Autism is characterized by immune system dysfunctions, social withdrawal, anxiety, irritability, seizures, loss of speech, lack of eye contact, extreme sensitivities, involuntary flapping and jerking motions, poor IQ or mental retardation, head banging, and sleep issues—symptoms that bear a striking resemblance to those seen in cases of mercury poisoning.[7]

With the population's increasing exposure to mercury and other chemicals in our food, water, air, and products, the possibility of a connection between environmental toxins and autism cannot be ignored. Until now, the search for answers regarding the rising autism epidemic has focused almost entirely on looking for genetic causes, and the focus makes sense. Autism Spectrum Disorder (ASD), a continuum of psychological conditions characterized by inhibited social functioning and repetitive behavior,[8] snakes through family trees, touching a brother, an uncle, a daughter in different generations, one with symptoms so severe he can't tie his shoes, count to ten, or look you in the eyes, who reacts with screaming terror to a shower and must live his adult life under constant care; another with Asperger's syndrome, prone to obsessions, with an eerily precise memory and few friends, but able to hold a job and buy a house—what's known in autism circles as "high functioning."

"Scientists Have the Genetic Causes of Autism in Their Sights," cheered a June 9, 2010, headline in *The Guardian*.[9] The findings of the Autism Genome Project, for which more than 120 scientists from nineteen countries pored over the genetic blueprints of people with autism from nearly 1,200 families with at least two members with autism— had just been published in the journal *Nature*.[10] Like science detectives on the trail of a mystery, they found clues: people with autism were more likely to have extra pieces or missing pieces in their genetic codes, what are known as copy number variations—some inherited from the parents, some unique to the child. The research highlighted new places where autism may be hiding, pointing to parts of the genetic code that determine how brains are wired and how brain cells communicate with one another. A press release from the National Institute of Mental Health (NIMH), which funded the study along with the group Autism Speaks, stated, "Autism likely stems from faulty wiring."[11] In other words, something happened when the brain cells of children with autism were formed, some interruption or interference that left them with perpetually missed signals. But the genetic discoveries of the well-funded, comprehensive Autism Genome Project could only explain 3 percent of autism cases.[12]

The search for environmental triggers for autism turned a major corner in July 2011 with the release of the California Autism Twins Study.[13] It was the first time that researchers had not only identified identical and fraternal twins with autism based on existing medical or parental reports, but had vigorously confirmed autism diagnoses in every case using "structured clinical assessments by both parental interview and direct child observation."[14] Twins offer an ideal way for researchers to assess how much of a disease or disorder is genetic, since identical twins have the exact same genetic makeup and fraternal twins share 50 percent of genes. In this case, researchers assessed 192 twin pairs representing diverse socioeconomic backgrounds born in California between 1987 and 2004, each of which included at least one twin with autism. Seventy-seven percent of male identical twins both had an ASD, and 31 percent of male fraternal twins. Among female twins, just 50 percent of identical twins both had the disorder, and 36 percent of fraternal twins. Mathematical modeling led the researchers to conclude that environmental factors—which were not specifically named— played a larger role than genetic heritability in the majority of autism cases. Heritability, they found, could account for 38 percent of ASD cases, while a "shared twin environmental component" accounted for 58 percent of cases. The report concluded, "Although genetic factors also play an important role, they are of substantially lower magnitude than estimates from prior twin studies of autism."

Other researchers are looking beyond genetics to a field called epigenetics, which means, literally translated, "over" or "above" genetics. It's been called the ghost in our genes, the hidden influence that makes our brain cells, or our heart cells, uniquely ours. All the cells in the body start out with the exact same genetic information. But some cells will go on to be liver cells, or heart cells, or brain cells. As Dr. Shuk-Mei Ho, chair of environmental health at the University of Cincinnati says, "epigenetics are the means or ways that the cell can petition the genome, the cell, into its active and inactive components [so that] some cells will become a heart cell, some cells will become a neuron" and so on.[15] Epigenetics turns specific genes "on" or "off", and can be influenced by almost anything—environmental toxins, poor dietary choices, drugs, stress. Epigenomes don't change the DNA—the genome—itself, but leave a lasting impression.

Dr. Ho says, "epigenetics is the link, the connector, between the environment and the genome."[16] It's also the most exciting avenue of research connected to autism—and the most sci-fi. With epigenetics, there's some evidence that your life experiences and dietary habits can impact not only your own gene expression, but that of your future grandkids and great grandkids. In a 2005 study looking at a remote Swedish village, researchers made a startling revelation. It appeared that grandfathers born in the nineteenth century who lacked sufficient access to food before puberty had grandsons with a longer life expectancy.[17] The grandsons had inherited some means of adapting that gave them an advantage genetics alone couldn't explain.

The latest research reinforces the idea that when it comes to autism, genetics can't tell the whole story. The July 2011 study from California indicated that in 58 percent of identical twin pairs, one sibling has autism and the other does not, despite the fact that they share identical genetic information.[18] Dr. Michael Merzenich, a neuroscientist, says: "Because autism is strongly inherited and because there is clearly an increase in incidence, the environmental factors that are contributing to the rise in incidence must be pretty widely out there in virtually almost every kid's environment."[19] There were 75.6 million children in the United States as of 2011.[20] According to the Centers for Disease Control and Prevention (CDC), an estimated 1 in 110 kids have ASD—that's about 690,000 total.

And the rate of cases is climbing rapidly with no sign of abating. In the most recent CDC study of autism in the US, looking at the prevalence of the disorder among eight-year-olds in eleven states— Alabama, Arizona, Colorado, Florida, Georgia, Maryland, Missouri, North Carolina, Pennsylvania, South Carolina, and Wisconsin—the agency found that rates went up 57 percent between 2002 and 2006. Boys were 4.5 times as likely to have the disorder as girls.[21] Autism has rocketed to the top of the long list of childhood disorders, diseases, and sensitivities on the rise, and will be diagnosed for more children in a given year than cancer, diabetes, and AIDS combined.[22]

Dr. Suruchi Chandra, a psychiatrist with the True Health Medical Center outside of Chicago who treats children with autism, said in a teleconference on autism and toxic chemicals in June 2011 that if the rise in autism numbers were due only to improved diagnosis and awareness of autism among the medical community—if the root of the epidemic were primarily genetic—she and other professionals would have seen an increase in adult or adolescent patients who had not been diagnosed, or had been misdiagnosed, in the past. But that is not the case. Rather, she said, "We're seeing an increase in the rates of ASDs in children. Really, only children." Another presenter, Dr. Irva Hertz-Picciotto, an environmental epidemiologist with the Medical Investigation of Neurodevelopmental Disorders (MIND) Institute at the University of California, Davis, went on to say, "The genes, it's become clear more and more, are not going to explain the whole story. What seems to be especially critical is the prenatal environment and potential interaction between susceptibility genes and environmental chemicals."[23]

Their research suggests that most people with autism have a genetic predisposition that has been exploited by chemical exposure, particularly during the highly vulnerable first trimester when a fetus' brain rapidly forms. Consider what happens during this incredible process.

Between the third and fourth week of pregnancy, the baby's brain begins to take shape, and the neural tube connecting the brain to the spinal cord closes; by the fifth week, the brain's hemispheres start to form. During the nine months that the baby is growing inside the womb, his brain is generating about 250,000 neurons per minute. By the time he is born, his brain will contain around 100 billion neurons. Even beyond toddlerhood, the human brain is a work in progress; the dendrites, or branches, of some neurons can continue to grow into old age.[24] Any chemical interruption in this incredibly complex process can change the way cells divide and synapses form, leaving a debilitating impact on a child's later development and impeding his ability to learn, speak, and socialize.

The idea that a toxin can cause autism is neither controversial nor speculative. Certain drugs, when taken during pregnancy, are already known to cause autism: the sedative thalidomide, used in the 1960s to treat morning sickness, was definitively tied to the later development of autism in children in 1994; valproic acid, an anticonvulsant used to treat mania and bipolar disorders, was also linked to autism beginning in 1994; and misoprostol, a drug used to control ulcers, disrupts a fetus' normal neural development and was found to give rise to autism in 2001.[25] In addition, an organophosphate insecticide called chlorpyrifos, used widely in homes to control cockroaches, has been tied to pervasive developmental disorder (PDD), a form of autism.[26] And a Swedish study from 2002 found that mothers who smoked regularly during early pregnancy were 40 percent more likely to give birth to a child with autism.[27]

Many other chemicals distributed far and wide across the natural world by power plant smokestacks, leaking waste sites, improper storage facilities, and outdated manufacturing processes have been proven to cause injury to developing brains. Lax chemical policies allow chemicals to circulate freely in our homes, products, and food supply, even though their health impacts have not been tested. These include mercury, lead, and polychlorinated biphenyls (PCBs); manmade organic chemicals used in electrical equipment, insulation, plastic, and a host of other materials; chemicals found in certain pesticides used in the home and sprayed on pets; organic solvents like toluene (found in paint thinners, car exhaust, and nail polish) and styrene (used in boatbuilding); polybrominated diphenyl ethers (PBDEs), flame retardants used in furniture foam, electronics, TV cabinets, and computer plastics; and phthalates, a group of plasticizers so ubiquitous that just one kind—di-(20ethylhexyl) phthalate or DEHP—is produced at the rate of four billion pounds per year in the US alone.[28]

Until recently, the controversy surrounding a possible connection between autism and the heavy metals present in vaccines has all but drowned out a more comprehensive look at these potentially problematic chemicals present in our food, air, water, products, and prescribed drugs. Andrew Wakefield, the British researcher responsible for drawing the vaccine connection to autism, was discredited for using unethical methods and accepting a £50,000 payout to tailor his findings.[29] Although no evidence of harm was ever discovered, the mercury-containing preservative thimerosal was removed from or reduced in all vaccinations for children six and under with the exception of the flu vaccine beginning in 2001.[30] It is now understood that a tuna sandwich contains more mercury[31] than a typical vaccine dose,[32] and that thimerosal in fact contains ethyl mercury, which has a shorter half-life than tuna's methylmercury.[33] Parents are not wrong to be concerned about heavy metals and other toxic chemicals that cause neurological damage when trying to make sense of a child's autism diagnosis, but they have largely been looking in the wrong place for those toxic exposures.

More than 80,000 chemicals are registered for use in the US,[34] 3,000 of which the Environmental Protection Agency (EPA) has classified as high production volume (HPV), meaning they are produced at a rate of more than one million pounds per year. Some 43 percent of these HPV chemicals have not been tested for basic toxicity, and 80 percent of them have not been tested for developmental toxicity, or how they will affect a developing fetus.[35] Companies are not required to disclose every ingredient on the back labels of spray cleaners or detergents, and only warn you if it's poisonous, dangerous, or may cause burns.[36] Without testing data, there's little to guide parents making cost-conscious decisions in supermarket aisles; most don't have the time to worry how many parts per billion (ppb) of a particular toxic chemical represents acceptable exposure.

The National Toxicology Program's website assures us that, despite the lack of testing for thousands of HPV chemicals, there is nothing to worry about. They write: "We do not know the effects of many of these chemicals on our health, yet we may be exposed to them while manufacturing, distributing, using, and disposing of them or when they become pollutants in our air, water, or soil. Relatively few chemicals are thought to pose a significant risk to human health."[37] Of course, without any relevant data, it's hard to take comfort in such breezy assurances.

Fortunately, researchers looking for ways to curb the staggering number of autism cases worldwide are conducting the investigations that federal agencies have failed to require of chemical manufacturers. With the exception of lead and cotinine (found in tobacco), studies of the number and amounts of chemicals that have taken up residence in our bodies by testing blood, urine, and other samples—known as biomonitoring studies—are fairly new. The National Health and Nutrition Examination Survey, administered by the CDC, didn't include a test to measure pollutant levels in the body until 1999,[38] but since that time CDC scientists have tested for the presence of 219 chemicals in study participants' blood or urine. The study has shown that the US population's exposure to industrial chemicals and heavy metals like mercury is on the rise; some chemical exposures are so ubiquitous that nearly every participant has registered detectable levels in his or her blood or urine. In the 2004 study, one type of PBDE was present in nearly everyone studied. BPA, a chemical used in the epoxy lining of canned foods, in certain plastic products, and on store receipts, was found in more than 90 percent of urine samples. Nearly every participant had measurable levels of perfluorooctanoic acid (PFOA), a chemical byproduct of nonstick coatings used in cookware. While children's blood lead levels have dropped dramatically since studies first began in the 1970s, total blood mercury levels measured between 1999 and 2004 have increased with age for all groups.[39]

Children, who are more vulnerable to the health impacts—from reproductive problems to learning disabilities—have higher levels of chemicals in their bodies than their parents, and researchers are finding that exposures to many common chemicals and heavy metals raise the likelihood of giving birth to a child with autism. Biomonitoring studies by Environmental Working Group (EWG) and other collectives of concerned individuals have found an average of 200 pollutants in the umbilical cord blood of infants, including mercury from tainted fish supplies, dental fillings, and the air surrounding coal-burning power plants; pesticides sprayed on crops, as well as in the home; flame retardants in computer and electronic equipment, mattresses, and other household goods; PCBs in plastic products and vinyl flooring; perfluorinated compounds (PFCs) in meat, fish, and dairy products;[40] PBDEs in breast milk;[41] and BPA in canned foods, food-storage containers, baby bottles, reusable water bottles, and receipts.[42] Contrary to the NTP's claim, the large majority of these industrial chemicals are implicated in dangerous health impacts, including cancer, brain and nervous system damage, reproductive health problems, and birth defects. Among administered drugs, antidepressants[43] and labor-inducing pitocin[44] are both suspects in rising autism numbers.

Dr. Philip Landrigan, director of the Children's Environmental Health Center at Mount Sinai School of Medicine in New York, became something of a celebrity in children's health circles when his early work connecting lead exposure with lowered IQ in children led to the banning of lead components from paint and gasoline. As a result, children's blood lead levels have declined by 80 percent since the late 1970s.[45] He has turned his focus to finding a connection between autism and environmental toxins, stating that we are in a "time of crisis," and our population's exposure to thousands of untested chemicals has essentially made our children the subjects of a "massive toxicological experiment."[46]

Landrigan, who resembles a stylish grandfather—trim white hair and mustache, intense blue eyes and an easy smile—is skilled at translating chemical- and medical-speak for lay audiences. His many fans and supporters hope he can help uncover the combination of chemicals driving the autism epidemic, so that those chemicals, too, will be cast out, relics of an earlier time when highly toxic chemicals were treated with innocent abandon—a time when no one thought twice about scrubbing the house with bleach and ammonia, smoking cigarettes in the bedroom, or rolling mercury across the table.

ONE

Uncounted Numbers
Urban Exposures, Chemical Concentrations,
and the Question of Race

Thanks to years of public health campaigns and plenty of media cover-age, many people are aware that certain types of fish are contaminated by mercury. Mercury released through emissions from coal-burning power plants and municipal and medical waste incinerators takes to the air and is carried along, sometimes for miles, before settling in soil or water. The inorganic mercury is absorbed into microorganisms in the water and converted to an organic substance, methylmercury, which is then consumed by fish. Big fish like shark, swordfish, king mackerel, and tilefish eat small, contaminated fish and accumulate high concen-trations of toxic methylmercury. Both white (albacore) and canned light tuna contain mercury, too, with a January 2011 investigation from *Consumer Reports* finding that "children and women of childbearing age can easily consume more mercury than the Environmental Protec-tion Agency considers advisable simply by eating one serving [about 2.5 ounces] of canned white tuna or two servings of light tuna per week."[1]

Women who eat large quantities of such fish, both during and after pregnancy, can readily pass that mercury on to infants through umbilical cord blood[2] and through their breast milk.[3] Pregnant women exposed to methylmercury from fish—particularly canned fish—have shown a greater likelihood for giving birth prematurely,[4] and a child born with low birth weight (4.4 pounds or less), such as happens when babies are born premature, is five times as likely to be diagnosed with autism as a child born at normal weight.[5] Recognizing that mercury from seafood "may harm an unborn baby or young child's developing nervous system," the Food and Drug Administration (FDA) has advised women to limit their consumption of certain fish while pregnant.[6]

Knowing of these dangers, many women choose not to eat fish high in mercury during pregnancy. But most populations exposed to toxic chemicals are not made aware that their food, water, or air could be poisonous. The likelihood of chemical exposure is deeply intertwined with a community's socioeconomic status; factories that spew pollution are often allowed to operate with impunity alongside poor communities whose residents aren't given the choice to opt out by simply avoiding contaminated items.

An early example of what can occur when factories pollute unchecked happened in Minamata, Japan, a small village of rice farmers and fishermen who depended on fish and shellfish from the Minamata Bay and the Shiranui Sea. In 1907 the Chisso Corporation opened a carbide plant on the shores of the bay. The townspeople initially welcomed the factory with the hope that it would bring economic prosperity. In 1930 the Chisso factory turned its attentions to the production of materials that could be used for Japan's growing military needs—specifically acetaldehyde, or ethanol, a needed energy source for a country without its own oil supplies, and polyvinyl chloride (PVC), which was used for airplane parts. As the factory rapidly expanded its production, it dumped increasing amounts of untreated waste into local water supplies, contaminating the bay and the sea with methylmercury from 1932 to 1968. As the chemical bioaccumulated in the local fish and shellfish, widespread mercury poisoning—Minamata disease, as it came to be called—seeped into the village.

It was the cats they noticed first—acting crazy, falling into the sea, as if they were committing suicide. The first official case of Minamata disease was recorded in 1956, when two sisters, ages five and two, exhibited symptoms that included convulsions, muscle contractions, twisting and repetitive movements of the hands and feet, and sudden screaming fits. They were determined to have an unknown disease of the central nervous system. Soon researchers from Kumamoto University discovered that many residents living around Minamata Bay showed an inability to grasp small objects and difficulty with hearing, seeing, walking, running, and swallowing. Once the symptoms began, they could progress within weeks to massive convulsions, insanity, coma, and death.[7] A black-and-white image of a mother and child known as "La Pieta de Minamata" has come to symbolize the heartbreak. The mother's head is wrapped in a scarf, her shoulders bare, her face lit ethereally, as she cradles and bathes her profoundly disabled child. The child looks, in fact, to be a young man, his neck muscles strained, legs and arms shortened and deformed, hands shriveled and bent.

The National Institute for Minamata Disease reports that as of 2001 there have been nearly 3,000 certified patients with the disease—some 1,784 of whom have died—and more than 10,000 with "applicable conditions such as sensory disorders or a high consumption of marine products."[8] Not until April 2006, nearly fifty years from the first report of the disease, did sufferers and their caregivers receive a formal apology from Prime Minister Junichiro Koizumi for the Japanese government's failure to stop the pollution. Many victims are still fighting legal battles for compensation.[9]

The Minamata tragedy was clearly linked to the Chisso factory, but it is often difficult to pin symptoms and diseases on exposure to chemicals from one particular source. People living in highly polluted urban areas are subject to a host of environmental contaminants that can lead to preterm birth. Pregnant mothers are more likely to give birth prematurely , or give birth to babies who are small for their gestational age, when they live near highways and are exposed to the associated air pollution, including carbon monoxide, nitrogen dioxide, sulfur dioxide and particulate matter.[10]

Sharon Sandifer-Holmes, a special education teacher who has several family members with autism, grew up with six siblings in a crowded apartment in an African-American community in the Bronx. There, environmental contamination was a constant presence, from the smog to the rusted pipes to the peeling lead paint in her mom's pre-war high rise, a subtler type of toxic exposure to which Sharon and her family never gave a second thought. But lead dust rises to the surface of lead paint and ends up on the floor, where children can easily ingest it in the normal course of crawling and putting objects in their mouths. Lead exposure is strongly linked to problems with cognitive functioning, including impaired learning and memory, mental retardation and developmental delay, psychiatric disturbances, seizures, and pre-term delivery.[11] Dr. Mark Mitchell, the founder and president of the Connecticut Coalition for Environmental Justice (CCEJ), a group that works to educate urban communities about existing pollutants and to give those communities a say before new polluting industries are ushered in, notes that "If you rent your own housing, you don't have control over when it's painted or how it's painted. . . . So children are much more likely to be exposed to chipping and peeling paint."[12]

Sharon was the one to take care of her youngest brother when it became clear he had severe autism. Six years older than her brother, she took on the role of teaching him as much as she could—how to say the alphabet and count to ten, how to tie his shoes. She learned to brush off the inevitable stares that followed her brother whenever they were out in public. Now in his midthirties, and with their mother no longer able to care for him at home, Sharon's brother is in a home for special needs adults full-time. Sharon's aunt and her nephew—both of whom were born and raised in the Bronx—also have autism.

Still living in the same apartment, Sharon gave birth to a son, James. In 1997 James failed to meet early milestones like walking and talking, but despite her familiarity with the signs of autism, Sharon didn't immediately make the connection. James was born seven weeks early, so Sharon assumed her son would be a little behind developmentally; she didn't know that premature birth is a risk factor for autism.[13] But the difference between James and other kids his age grew too pronounced to ignore. He didn't start walking until he was thirteen months old. He didn't look his mother in the eyes, or show her any affection. "I was like, 'Wow, something is not right here," Sharon says. "Plus the fact that it was in my family, the light bulb went off in my head. I'm like, 'I need to get him checked. I need to get out of that denial stage and take the first step.'"[14] She made an appointment for James at the Kennedy Child Study Center in the Bronx, where they confirmed that he had PDD, a catchall term that means James showed severe impairments in thinking, language, affection, and social interaction. In other words, he is autistic.

By the time James turned six, Sharon had fallen in love and was pregnant with her second son, Chris. She moved to Bridgeport, Connecticut to live with her husband, affectionately known as "Big Chris." They live on a quiet, tree-lined street in one of a string of brick townhouses with matching white awnings not far from the former Remington Arms Factory. Flowering bushes and a pinwheel or two brighten the small, fenced front yards. It's quiet here, and the neighbors are neighborly. For Sharon, Bridgeport is an improvement over the crowded Bronx apartment. But the Bridgeport Harbor Station—a coal-burning power plant that burns 997,370 tons of coal per year and is located between the city's downtown and South End neighborhoods—produces over 3,000,000 tons of carbon dioxide emissions per year according to 2006 data, along with over 2,000 tons of nitrogen oxide emissions, nearly 3,000 tons of sulfur dioxide emissions, and 54 pounds of mercury.[15] Families like Sharon's living within a mile of the plant have an average income of just $11,400, and 87 percent of those living in the plant's vicinity are people of color. Jacqui Patterson of the National Association for the Advancement of Colored People (NAACP) Climate Justice Initiative took a walking tour of the Bridgeport Harbor Station and its surrounding neighborhoods in April 2010 and reported seeing "the highest mountain of coal" she'd seen in her many visits to urban coal plants; it was left uncovered and resulted in a film of coal dust over her car. Residents reported the same coal dust regularly coated their cars and kept them from opening their windows or hanging out their laundry.[16]

The coal-burning power plant is just one of many toxic burdens the city's largely poor and minority urban residents must bear. An aerial map of the city shows it dotted, chicken pox-like, with brownfield sites—abandoned parcels of former industrial land that are now polluted—208 of them with leaking underground storage tanks. The massive thoroughfare of I-95, which bisects the city, sends nearly 130,000 cars and trucks barreling through Bridgeport each day as they pass between New York City to the south and Boston to the north.[17] Meanwhile, Bridgeport RESCO Company, a waste-to-energy plant on the city's west side, has failed to monitor for heavy metal emissions in the past, burning a massive pile of construction debris called "Mount Trashmore" between 1992 and 1993 that included asbestos and toxic metals "without extra monitoring of air emissions."[18]

"In Bridgeport, you can have industrial facilities in the middle of a residential block," says Dr. Mitchell of the CCEJ. "It was set up originally so people could work where they live and they could walk to work [one of hundreds of city factories producing items such as sewing machines, brass parts, Frisbie pies, gramophones, and corsets]. But because of the toxicity of industries, it's not workable any more. There needs to be a buffer. So in many places in the 1920s, the zoning started moving toward separating the residential from the commercial. But other cities didn't. Bridgeport is one of them."[19] At a former chrome plating facility in Bridgeport, Dr. Mitchell saw children playing inside an abandoned building where they could be exposed to chromium 6, a serious toxin associated with cancer, skin ulcers, and kidney damage.

In the city's north end sits the sprawling remains of the Remington Complex—the former GE arms factory, composed of thirteen interconnected buildings five stories high spread across more than seventy-six acres. Once, it was the largest munitions manufacturer in the world.[20] Now, the decrepit, blackened brick buildings with broken windows and rusted metal balconies are stacked like giant, duplicate Lego structures, devoid of activity—unless you count the rumored ghostly presence of workers who lost their lives there in molten metal accidents and deadly explosions.[21] Hazardous wastes produced at the plant were initially stored onsite in leaky drums containing cyanide, mercury, and PCBs.[22]

Could a child's risk for developing autism be tied to exposure to such persistent environmental toxins? One study looking at autism cases in San Francisco found a substantial link between mothers living in areas of high environmental air pollutants and their likelihood of having children with autism. The researchers matched the health records for children born in 1994 in six counties in San Francisco—284 of whom had autism—with relevant pollution data. Where environmental air pollutants including heavy metals like mercury, cadmium and nickel; industrial solvents like trichloroethylene (or trichloroethene, TCE, used to clean metal parts); and gases like vinyl chloride (used to make PVCs, which are in many plastic pipes, wires and packaging materials) were highest, the risk factor for autism increased by 50 percent.[23] The hazardous air pollutants studied came from sources as varied as car, plane, train and ship emissions; dry cleaners, gas stations, and large industrial manufacturing facilities; and home cleaning products.

The Agency for Toxic Substances and Disease Registry (ATSDR) and the EPA are required to maintain a list of substances from industrial facilities that pose the greatest threats to human health. The entire list contains a whopping 276 priority hazardous chemicals.[24] Mercury is ranked third behind arsenic and lead in terms of frequency, toxicity and potential for human exposure. Vinyl chloride ranks fourth. In the San Francisco study, subjects were exposed to so many overlapping chemicals that researchers were unable to tease apart data linking individual chemicals with autism rates. Instead, they categorized compounds as either metals or solvents. They were also unable to take into account the subjects' personal habits, such as smoking or eating contaminated food. However, they concluded that, as such limitations in exposure estimates are "unlikely to vary by case status, the effect estimates are probably shifted toward the null."[25]

This was not the first study to link higher autism rates with environmental toxins, specifically exposure to heavy metals. A 2004 study in Texas found that for every 1,000 pounds of environmentally released mercury, there was a 43 percent increase in the rate of special education services and a 61 percent increase in the rate of autism.[26] Children in urban districts were found to be particularly at risk for autism; relative to rural districts, urban districts showed a 473 percent higher rate of autism. Suburban districts had a 255 percent higher rate of autism compared to their rural counterparts.[27]

And stress makes people more vulnerable to toxic assaults. Black mothers are more likely to be affected by the stress of struggling to make a living than white mothers. One 2006 study relating particulate exposure to low-birth-weight babies reported in the journal *Pediatrics* that among Georgia mothers who participated in the study, there were 69 infants born preterm—31.9 percent of these infants were born to white mothers, 68.1 percent of them were born to non-white mothers.[28] Another study in the *American Journal of Epidemiology* analyzing race, neighborhood deprivation (neighborhoods whose residents exhibit low incomes, high unemployment rates, and a tendency not to finish high school) and preterm births reported 2004 vital statistics data showing that 13.7 percent of infants born to black mothers were low birth weight, compared to 7.2 percent for white mothers, with factors like income, education and housing playing a significant role. The study went on to note that "Preterm birth . . . is responsible for two thirds of infant deaths and approximately half of subsequent childhood neurologic problems in the United States." Even when researchers control for factors like maternal smoking, the racial disparity in preterm birth rates remains, leading researchers to conclude that larger neighborhood factors, such as living conditions and the stressors of poverty, racism, violence, and exposure to toxins and contaminants, are at play.[29]

One of the lead researchers who looked at neighborhood deprivation and preterm births, Dr. Patricia O'Campo, says those affected have a lifetime of issues ahead. "Babies born early have a high risk of subsequent adverse developmental health problems," O'Campo says. "And a whole lot can happen between giving birth and when a child is assessed with interventions."[30] A premature baby literally has less brain matter evident at ages seven to fifteen than his or her carried-to-term counterpart; and males are "most vulnerable to adverse neurodevelopmental outcomes."[31] But recent studies have revealed something else about such infants: if early interventions and innovative teaching programs are applied—if a parent knows about such services and has access to them—the child can develop normally and succeed in school.[32] Women living in low-income, toxic, and high-stress environments, then, are at a double disadvantage, with both an increased likelihood to give birth to babies prematurely, and less access to the services that can improve their child's development when it is most critical. "There's a lot of recent information about psycho-social stress and toxins," Mitchell says. "Hundreds of studies [have been] done. If you live in a bad neighborhood, the stress from racism, the stress from poverty. Poverty is not nearly as important as the inequality of income. So if you make much less than the people around you than that's much more stressful than if everybody were poor. If you live in a drug-infested neighborhood, if you're exposed to a certain level of toxins, your body will have more of a reaction to the toxins than if you don't have the stress level."[33]

A poor city could hardly be more juxtaposed with wealthy neighbors than Bridgeport, Connecticut's most populous city, where more than 70 percent of residents are black and Hispanic, and 20 percent live in poverty.[34] Meanwhile, Fairfield, Connecticut, just over the border, was ranked in the top ten best places to live by CNN's *Money Magazine*,[35] thanks to its five beaches, high-performing schools, low crime, upscale restaurants, and winding, leafy streets that showcase one perfectly manicured lawn after another. Passing through it on I-95, Bridgeport's visible cityscape offers little to welcome potential visitors but empty brick warehouses, a belching smokestack, and vacant lots. Its small downtown, a collection of historic bank buildings and storefronts from a more prosperous era, is eerily lifeless at night despite lofty ambitions for revitalization from each subsequent city administration.

Bridgeport is similar to many cities across the country where minority residents live with a daily onslaught of chemical exposures from power plant smokestacks, contaminated factories, and outdated school buildings; from highways and congested streets; and from old apartment high rises where walls and windows still contain lead paint. For Sharon, those exposures would have been most worrisome when she lived in the Bronx, during the time when she was pregnant and first raising her infant son. But the Bronx could just as easily have been Chicago's Pilsen or Little Village neighborhoods, each home to an outdated coal-burning power plant that together (as of 2009) release 90 pounds of mercury and 265 pounds of lead per year into surrounding densely populated communities;[36] or Houston, Texas, which boasts some of the most consistently polluted air in the country thanks to major traffic and a concentration of chemical industry and power plants;[37] or Pittsburgh, Pennsylvania; Birmingham, Alabama; Detroit, Michigan; Los Angeles, California—all of which rank among the most polluted cities in the US with record levels of air pollution and particle emissions.[38]

Sharon works for a Bridgeport public elementary school with kids who have a range of learning disabilities, including autism and attention deficit hyperactivity disorder (ADHD), and emotional problems. She sees that many city kids are not getting diagnosed early enough—often not until they are twelve or thirteen, according to their individualized education plans, which are used to define shortcomings and differentiate instruction for special needs kids. The children need services they aren't getting. Mostly, she says, the parents don't know what to do or are in denial. "They just think their kids are going through something and they'll grow out of it," Sharon says.

Since Sharon took care of her autistic brother and works with autistic children, she has an advantage over most parents of autistic children. Looking back, Sharon realizes her son was likely having small seizures in his sleep around the age of twelve, because when James woke in the morning his tongue would be chewed on either side. But it wasn't confirmed until she received a phone call from the bus driver one morning that James had had a small seizure. After that, the seizures came with more frequency and intensity. The spasms lasted less than a minute, but they occured several times a day. One day, he had five seizures in the span of twenty-four hours. When James first experienced multiple seizures, Sharon rushed him to the emergency room where he was kept overnight and administered medicines intravenously. Now he visits a neurologist every three months, and since starting anti-seizure medications, including Topomax and Trileptal, has improved.[39]

Inside the family's home is a coffee-colored sectional couch with a large matching ottoman. When James comes downstairs, he pauses by the ottoman, rubbing the corner. After walking by, he changes direction, so he can touch the ottoman again. When he's uncomfortable, he makes high, whining noises, grabs his ear repeatedly and looks away from the person speaking to him. He rocks in place. But when his mom asks James about his notes, he becomes excited, talking in a flurry of words, proud, suddenly, and forgetting for a moment that there's a stranger in the room. James loves to write notes; every day, over and over, he writes a note to the woman with a little boy who lives across the street—a family he's never officially met. The note reads, "Dear lady from 312, for Christmas I want potato chips, Frosted Flakes, chicken nuggets." "He'll write the note fifty times a day," Sharon says, "and the note will say the same thing all of the times." When James comes home from school, he runs up to his mother, nearly bursting, saying, "Mom, mom, this is what I wrote for you at school, guess what I wrote?" And Sharon unfolds the note and reads: "Dear Mom, for Christmas I want . . ."

Sharon's ability to recognize the warning signs for autism early meant that James has been able to get the help—both at school and from doctors—that will allow him to steadily become more capable and communicative and to overcome life-threatening complications like seizures. That's not always the case, particularly in urban districts. The signs of autism are often present from birth: the child isn't making eye contact or responding to his name, he's not babbling by age one, not playing with toys, and seems not to hear. But as Sharon has noticed in the schools where she's taught—where the large majority of students are black and Hispanic, where all kids qualify for free meals and many homes are run by a single parent—a parent not aware of these signs can miss out on critical early intervention.

Black children, according to one study, are being diagnosed with autism an average of 1.4 years later than white children when they are brought in for testing, losing valuable treatment time.[40] When researchers looked at groups of families on Medicaid in relation to how autism was diagnosed, they found that black children were nearly three times more likely to receive another diagnosis on their first visit to a specialist. Most often, they were instead deemed to have conduct or hyperactivity disorder. And a family's insurance status plays a role, too. Those who had been on Medicaid for more than a year, as opposed to less than a year, were 3.4 times as likely to receive a diagnosis other than autism.[41]

When the CDC looked at rising autism numbers nationwide in 2006, it found that the median age for autism diagnosis was between four and five years old, despite the fact that the kids in question showed concerning developmental shortcomings prior to age three. The finding prompted the CDC to launch an autism-related public awareness campaign called "Learn the Signs. Act Early."[42] Once a diagnosis has been made, school districts are required to provide services for special needs kids, including specialized education, or, if that is not available, to bus kids to schools with the necessary services. The Individuals with Disabilities Education Act (IDEA) does more than require these services—it works to ensure racial balance in the way such funds are distributed. However, since the law's inception in 1975, officials have noticed a troubling trend—black males, particularly those with behavioral problems, have been increasingly pushed into special education classrooms without an academic reason.[43] It is evident that minority communities need the tools both to recognize and describe their child's autism behaviors. Doctors, teachers, and specialists, for their part, should be more attuned to their own biases when it comes to diagnosing.

In the national autism conversation, the issue of race has been largely overlooked. Wendy Fournier, president of the National Autism Association, wrote that she's increasingly concerned about how autism has gone undiagnosed in minority communities, adding, "At the conferences we go to, there are no black people there, no minorities. It's kind of freaky."[44]

From celebrity advocates like the much-quoted actress Jenny McCarthy, whose child has autism, to promotional materials for leading autism groups, the face of autism is overwhelmingly white. The perceived imbalance has helped fuel the notion that the rise in autism reflects a parental and media hysteria, not an actual increase. That notion appeared to be vindicated by a California study in January 2010 in which researchers looked at the birth records of some 2.5 million babies born in California between 1996 and 2000, 10,000 of whom were later diagnosed with an ASD. Rather than finding clusters of autism cases around areas of high pollution and toxicity, researchers uncovered the opposite: autism cases in the state were clustered in the wealthiest cities and suburbs, places like San Francisco, Modesto,

Mission Viejo, and Beverly Hills, and Thousand Oaks in Los Angeles.[45] These are places where home values regularly exceed half a million dollars, and where residents are largely wealthy, white, and educated. The media response to the University of California, Davis study was immediate: environmental causes, it was reported, had little to do with autism clusters. Rather, these were educated parents pushing for special services because they had access to specialists and the means to pay for them. As a result, children in these well-to-do neighborhoods had autism rates nearly double those of surrounding regions.

What was largely missing from the story and related commentaries was that these families seeking and receiving early autism diagnoses and treatment did so because they had the education and means to identify the disorder and get help for their children. Other families—particularly black, minority, and low-income families—did not. The study unwittingly highlighted the fact that families who needed services were not being screened, diagnosed, or treated. Recognizing the signs of autism begins with the parents. A follow-up study done in March 2010 confirmed that parental knowledge about how to identify autism and seek treatment was critical in getting children diagnosed. Diagnosis happened more often when parents talked to other parents familiar with autism and were referred to area specialists. The resources for treating autism are out there, but, reports the study, in order to obtain them, "parents have to recognize the behavioral symptoms of autism, identify and reach a physician capable of identifying autism, and learn how to navigate the complex world of state developmental service departments, school systems, and other service vendors. Obviously, this knowledge is achieved, not ascribed."[46]

As autism becomes more universally recognized—and de-stigmatized—the racial gap is closing. The CDC findings on autism rates reflect a greater prevalence for autism among white children, particularly boys, but they also point to steadily climbing numbers in black and Hispanic populations. Between 2002 and 2006, the numbers of white children with autism jumped 55 percent; among black children, 41 percent; and among Hispanic children, 91 percent. Arizona's numbers reflected the most significant jump in Hispanic kids with autism—144 percent—a result, researchers later surmised, of the state doing a better job at recognizing and diagnosing autism in a population that had been seriously under-diagnosed.[47] The latest study of autism prevalence conducted in a community in South Korea that relied on in-person screenings of all children between ages seven and twelve (55,266 in total) instead of simply counting how many kids were enrolled in special education classes found that numbers were much higher than previously estimated. Published in the *American Journal of Psychiatry* in September 2011, the study found that one in thirty-eight children, or 2.64 percent, had autism—and two-thirds of the children who met the criteria had not been diagnosed and remained in mainstream schools and classrooms.[48] Bennett Leventhal, one of the study's authors and deputy director of New York's Nathan Klein Institute for Psychiatric Research, said, "There's no reason to think that South Korea has more children with autism than anyplace else in the world."[49]

Autism is on the rise in immigrant populations as well. Dr. Daphne Keen, a developmental pediatrician consultant and senior lecturer at St. George's University of London, noticed that a disproportionate number of immigrant parents were coming to clinics with children on the autism spectrum. She began asking other colleagues in the UK and abroad about what she'd noticed, and they'd all seen similar trends. So Keen and other researchers launched a study, published in April 2010, that combed through UK data to see if they could connect the dots. They found that immigrant parents, specifically those who had migrated to the UK from the Caribbean and Africa, were giving birth to children with autism at much higher rates than children of non-immigrant parents. Among the 428 children studied during a six-year period, the risk of increase for autism in children of Caribbean immigrant parents was five times higher than for the general population. The children of black immigrant mothers were five times as likely to have autism as children in the general population; the same did not hold true for children of black mothers in the UK in general, showing that immigration was the critical factor.[50] There were also substantial increased risks for the children of Asian immigrants.

A study in the mid-1970s in Australia found that children of Greek and German immigrant parents were more likely to have autism. In the 1980s and 1990s, other studies found increased autism risks for children born to immigrants, particularly in Sweden. But this was the first time that researchers had the extensive population and health records to draw such definitive conclusions. Such disparities could not be explained by race; they could only be explained by environmental factors.[51] Immigrants were subject to unique stressors, such as social isolation and adjustment difficulties, and may also have been more susceptible to the particular toxins in their new home countries as a result of that increased stress. It's possible that epigenetics plays a role; a stressful event like immigrating to a foreign country could carry epigenetic consequences.

Because the findings are so new, the exact causes driving these higher autism numbers among immigrants is still unknown. But as in the San Francisco and Texas studies, there's strong evidence linking environmental contamination and higher rates of autism. However, since autism research relies on community health records, and accurate health records, in turn, are dependent on a family's access to and use of services, study results are often skewed. Until there is comprehensive nationwide screening for autism and universal early healthcare services, the rates of autism will continue to be under-diagnosed, misdiagnosed, or diagnosed late in poor and minority communities—the very communities most at risk for elevated levels of toxic exposures.

TWO

Foreign Bodies

How We All Became Carriers of Mercury, Triclosan, and Flame Retardants

Mercury is a toxic shape-shifter, presenting itself in three different forms. The kind workers are exposed to is elemental, or metal, mercury, which causes severe neurological damage when the odorless mercury fumes are inhaled. Breathing mercury is one of the most dangerous routes of exposure; some 80 percent of the inhaled mercury travels directly to the bloodstream from the lungs and then moves rapidly to the brain and kidneys, where it might remain for months. The ATSDR writes, "When metallic mercury enters the brain, it is readily converted to an inorganic form and is 'trapped' in the brain for a long time." Metallic mercury passes easily from a pregnant mother's bloodstream to that of her developing child. Over time, after it has done its damage, the mercury will pass from the body in feces and urine.[1]

The second form of mercury, inorganic mercury salts, was once used in laxatives, worming medications, and teething powders. Today, they are found in skin-lightening creams, some antibacterial products, and within the preservatives thimerosal and phenylmercuric nitrate, which are used in some prescription and over-the-counter medications, and, in the case of thimerosal, multi-dose flu vaccines. Mercury salts are also present as mercuric sulfide in some colored paints and the red coloring of tattoo dyes. In general, less than 10 percent of swallowed mercury salts are absorbed by the body, but in certain cases up to 40 percent can pass through the lining of the stomach and intestines. Mercury salts can also enter the body through the skin and settle in the kidneys, or pass from a mother to her baby during breastfeeding.[2]

Finally, there's methylmercury—inorganic mercury that has been converted, or methylated, by tiny organisms in the water like bacteria, phytoplankton, and fungi. Methylmercury is easily absorbed into tissues and is difficult for fish (and animals, including humans) to eliminate. The bigger and older the fish, the more methylmercury they contain. Mushrooms grown in contaminated soil absorb methylmercury, and plants like corn, wheat, and peas can absorb smaller amounts.[3]

Mercury exposure does not just affect industrial workers in factories. At home, kids can inhale metal mercury fumes from broken thermometers; at school, they can be exposed in science labs. Improper clean-up and spills from medical waste and dental offices can lead to exposure. The ATSDR writes that "Some types of polyurethane flooring used in schools [a type of flooring often found in school gymnasiums] may give off mercury vapors, especially when damaged." Children are more sensitive to the impacts of these vapors than adults, and their bodies take longer to process and excrete the dangerous metal. Because kids breathe faster than adults, they take in mercury vapors in larger doses; because they are small, they come in closer contact with the vapors emanating from the floor when playing or crawling.[4]

It's not entirely known how many of these mercury-containing floors are out there, but one manufacturer claims to have installed over 25 million pounds of polyurethane flooring with a mercury-containing top coat in US school gymnasiums over the past forty years.[5] When the state health departments tested the airborne concentrations in suspect schools, they found amounts ranging from .042 (in the breathing zone) to 1.6 micrograms per cubic meter ($\mu g/m^3$). Not until school administrators in the central suburb of Westerville, Ohio, were looking to install new gym floors did they realize the old flooring was leaching mercury and posing harm to exposed students. Materials with a mercury level exceeding .2 milligrams per liter are classified as hazardous waste with stringent disposal protocol, and five of nine school floorings that were torn up and headed to the dump in Westerville exceeded hazardous material status.[6]

State officials began testing for vapors within schools still containing these 3M Tartan brand floors and discovered that indoor air inside one elementary school gym contained mercury levels up to 1.6 micrograms per cubic meter. Rubber balls, floor mats, and stage curtains were tested in sealed bags, and these, too, were off-gassing mercury in amounts ranging from 2 to 9 micrograms per cubic meter. Technically, these mercury levels were still within the ATSDR's established "safe zone" for mercury exposure, though the schools opted to replace the flooring and gym equipment as a preventative measure. An "action level" for replacing contaminated products like gym balls begins at 10 micrograms of mercury per cubic meter, just over the level found for some toys and equipment in Westerville schools. The minimum risk level established for chronic inhalation of mercury vapors, meanwhile, is set by the ATSDR at .2 micrograms per cubic meter, 100 times less than levels at which exposed workers begin experiencing subtle neurological impacts like tremors. In a residential setting, however—or, in this case, a school—acceptable exposure levels are set higher, since 1 microgram per cubic meter of mercury vapor is considered safe. But even in their report, officials had to admit that "the full extent of human health effects from long-term exposure to low levels of mercury vapor in indoor air are not fully understood," that "children playing in the gymnasium are likely exerting themselves and thus are breathing heavier and most likely would have a greater exposure than a sedentary person," and that "the polymer flooring material breaks down with age, possibly leading to the release of increasing levels of mercury vapor into the air through time." Echoing the manufacturer's admission, they wrote that "mercury vapor levels associated with this flooring might reach levels as high as 22 μg/m³."[7] The long-term health impacts this elemental mercury may have had on the Ohio kids who were exposed may never be known. Unless there is a high concentrated exposure, as happened with Danbury's hatmakers or the women and children of Minamata, Japan, the effects are harder to trace, and they manifest over longer periods of time. And when it comes to autism, it's the cumulative effect of multiple toxic exposures that is of greatest concern.[8] School gymnasium floors are just one among many.

Property contaminated by mercury can also be converted to a school or even a day-care center before the site has been safely cleaned up. That happened in historic Franklinville, New Jersey, when a building that once manufactured mercury thermometers was converted in 2004 to a children's daycare called Kiddie Kollege, sparking national outrage. The abandoned property had been bought in foreclosure and leased to the daycare; the real estate broker later claimed he had misinterpreted environmental reports. Before Kiddie Kollege was shut down in 2006, more than thirty toddlers and the daycare staff were exposed to mercury levels that exceeded occupational health and safety exposure limits more than threefold in certain areas. In the first-floor area, where toddlers were kept, levels of airborne mercury were more than 550 times the standard. Mercury was also detected in 98 out of 100 material and wipe samples tested.[9] The exposure led to a class-action lawsuit by parents of enrolled children seeking $1 million in damages, in part to continue monitoring the children's health for any adverse impacts that might manifest in later years.[10] Meanwhile, Public Employees for Environmental Responsibility reports that there are an estimated "1,400 day-care centers in New Jersey located on or within 400 feet of a known toxic hazard."[11]

And that's just New Jersey. In one report on children's exposure to elemental mercury, the ATSDR detailed 843 mercury-related events from 2002 through 2006, 409 of which may have involved children (most involved broken thermometers or mishandled mercury-containing equipment); the National Poison Data System reported 30,891 calls made to poison control centers regarding children's exposure to mercury from broken thermometers between 2002 and 2006, and 6,396 calls regarding children's exposure to elemental mercury from other sources; and ten published reports from 1998 to 2004 involved mercury contamination with approximately 1,393 children exposed to amounts of mercury ranging from 9 to 701 milliliters. The worst exposures involved children stealing mercury stored in canisters or bottles at industrial sites or in school science labs, attracted to the unique silver liquid that forms shiny, round droplets as it disperses.[12]

Household exposures to mercury are most obvious when they are centered around a major spill. In 1989 a fifteen-year-old boy in Ohio and later his eleven-year-old sister were admitted to an area hospital with symptoms that included aches, irritability, muscle weakness, rash, sweating, tremors, insomnia, anorexia, and an inability to think clearly. They first diagnosed the boy with measles. Later, it was discovered that a previous tenant living in the family's apartment had spilled a significant amount of elemental mercury. Upon testing, mercury vapors in seven rooms were found ranging from 50-400 micrograms per cubic meter. Both children were diagnosed with acrodynia—a mercury-triggered disease most often seen in children—with neuropsychiatric impairment. Even after three months of treatment, the girl could only walk short distances with assistance due to the pervasive muscle weakness.[13]

Less toxic levels of household mercury could come from any number of sources. The CDC reports that mercury is "added into many household products, such as latex paints, adhesives, joint compounds, acoustical plates, and cleaning solutions." Complicating matters, the agency adds that "not all products that contain mercury are labeled as such,"[14] so it's up to parents to properly ventilate rooms when using paints or cleaning products and to hope for the best.

The case of the Ohio children exposed to spilled mercury is the extreme—the proof, writ large, of the devastating effects of mercury poisoning on a child's developing brain and body. But regular mercury exposure on a smaller scale, with less severe or obvious impairments that can manifest as autism and other learning disabilities, is accepted as normal by our federal agencies.[15] The Food and Drug Administration estimates that most people are exposed to about 3.5 micrograms of mercury per day on average, most of it in the form of methylmercury that comes from eating fish. It's also absorbed via dental fillings, which can release small amounts of mercury vapors over time that are then inhaled.[16] And the number of women with detectable levels of mercury in their blood is on the rise. In the 1999–2000 National Health and Nutrition Examination Survey, mercury was detected in the blood of 2 percent of women ages eighteen to forty-nine. By the 2005–2006 survey, mercury was found in 30 percent of women in this age group.[17] Dan R. Laks of UCLA, the researcher who made the connection, said that we are at a juncture as a society where "chronic mercury exposure has reached a critical level," where mercury, deposited in the human body, is now rapidly accumulating.[18] The fact that disorders like autism, which are specifically tied to breakdowns in brain formation and function that could be caused by such an exposure, are also on the rise, strikes Laks as the inevitable outcome.

Knowing that mercury is dangerous—and even taking steps to avoid exposure—cannot change the fact that we've got increasing amounts of this metal swimming through our bloodstreams, altering our development in many quiet, destructive ways. When the nonprofit Environmental Working Group decided to find out just how many chemicals were present in our bloodstreams, they went right to the source, taking samples of umbilical cord blood from ten babies born in different US hospitals. Once upon a time, the group writes in the study's introduction, scientists thought the mother's placenta acted as a de facto filter, shielding a developing fetus from harmful contaminants in her bloodstream or her environment. It turns out that's not the case. The cord blood they sampled contained an average of 200 industrial chemicals and pollutants, everything from mercury to pesticides to flame retardants to PCBs. All ten of the newborns had mercury in their bloodstreams, in concentrations ranging from .07 to 2.3 ppb.[19]

Professor James Adams, who runs the Autism/Asperger's Research Program at Arizona State University, began his career with a PhD in material science and engineering. But when his daughter, Kim, was diagnosed with autism in the late 1990s at age two and a half, he became frustrated with the lack of research looking at environmental causes for autism, and began his own search for answers. Adams was particularly interested in the mercury-autism connection. He began to study the baby teeth of children with autism, finding they contained twice as much mercury as did the teeth of non-autistic kids.[20] Adams's daughter's baby teeth had the second-highest mercury level in the study.[21] When Adams studied samples of the participants' hair (available from parents' baby scrapbooks), his findings were the opposite: children with autism had unusually low levels of mercury in their hair samples. The hair tests confirmed what the teeth tests had revealed: if autistic children were able to properly excrete mercury, it would be leaving their bodies through their hair; instead, the metal was building up to dangerous levels inside their bodies, including their teeth. Poring through medical records, Adams discovered another common thread. Children with autism had taken oral antibiotics 2.5 times as often as typical children during their first eighteen months, usually as a result of ear infections.[22] Antibiotics have a major impact on the way bodies—at least mice bodies—excrete mercury. One study from the 1980s looked at the difference in mercury retention between mice fed three different diets—pellets, evaporated milk, or a liquid (high protein/low fat) diet. The different diets did result in different mercury elimination half-times, which were 34, 10, and 5 days for mice fed milk, pellets and liquid diets respectively. But introduction of antibiotics during the experiments eliminated all dietary differences. "Under these conditions, the apparent Hg [mercury] elimination half-times were greater than 100 days regardless of the dietary regimen." Antibiotics, in other words, were inhibiting the animals' ability to get rid of mercury.[23] The recurring ear infections that prompted the treatments might also have signaled a deeper problem—something amiss with a child's immune system—but that was never explored. Adams says that today, "The two major sources [of mercury] are from dental fillings and seafood. And that in turn comes from the environment, from coal-burning power plants and other sources."[24]

Coal, which is rock made up of the remains of giant swampy plants that lived and died 100 to 400 million years ago, is buried in snaking lines known as seams hundreds of feet or more beneath the earth's surface. The seams, some of which are hundreds of feet thick, each represent hundreds or thousands of years of plant growth. These ancient plants absorbed mercury from the prehistoric air, so coal contains high levels of mercury that is released when it is burned.

Since this rich form of energy was discovered in the 1800s, humans have found increasingly innovative ways to get it out. Where coal is close enough to the surface, top layers are ripped out with bulldozers and power shovels. Where it's deep in the ground, workers descend down vertical shafts to extract it from as far as 1,000 feet beneath the earth. More recently, companies looking for faster ways to get at coal while employing the fewest people have turned to simply blasting off mountaintops with explosives in what's known as mountaintop removal mining. Thousands of blasts go off each day across the Appalachian Mountains—and anything that isn't coal is sent into the valleys below, choking and contaminating streams with rubble and debris and leaving ugly scars across the once-green mountains. Once collected, the coal is piled high in railroad cars and taken to power plants, where it's burned in boilers at about 1,000 degrees Farenheit, producing steam that's piped at high pressure into turbines that then spin generators to produce electricity. The thick smoke that rises from these plants' smokestacks contains particles of mercury and arsenic that settle across the land and sea.

Coal-burning power plants are the largest source of mercury emissions in the US, accounting for 50 percent of human-generated mercury emissions.[25] Technically, mercury is from the earth—it's an element of nature that humans cannot create or destroy—but by unearthing it in such large quantities and releasing it into the air, the harmless, inorganic mercury falls into the water and is absorbed into the tissues of fish and shellfish and converted into highly toxic methylmercury.

In 2000, the EPA launched a four-year study in which officials collected tissue samples from predator fish, such as bass and trout, and bottom-dwelling fish, such as carp and catfish. The fish were collected each year from the same 500 sites, selected at random from the 147,000 freshwater lakes and reservoirs in the lower forty-eight states. The samples were studied for 268 chemical residues, including mercury, pesticides, PCBs, and dioxins.

Scientists discovered PCBs (the production of which was banned in 1979) in every single fish taken from the 500 sampling sites. Mercury, too, was found in every fish tissue sample, and nearly half of the tissue samples—representing fish from more than 36,000 lakes—had mercury concentrations that exceeded the recommended 300 parts per billion limit designated as acceptable for human health. Among predator fish sampled, the highest mercury concentration found was an astonishing 6,605 ppb; in bottom-dwellers, the highest was 596 ppb.[26] Mercury is also the main reason states issue advisories related to catching and eating fish, and 80 percent of fish advisories issued in 2008 were at least partly due to mercury. In that year, more than 40 percent of the nation's total lake acreage was under advisory for mercury—that's approximately 18 million lake acres deemed unsafe for catching and eating fish.[27]

Coal-burning power plants are the biggest mercury-emitter in the US, but they're not the only ones. There are also outdated mercury chlorine, or chlor-alkali, plants, which produce mercury in the course of making chlorine gas and lye used for soap, detergent, plastic, and paper. Newer plants no longer use mercury, but older plants did. Thanks to efforts by nonprofit groups like Oceana, just two mercury-based chlorine plants have resisted upgrading their operations.[28] Mercury-based light switches in cars produce mercury vapors when they are melted and recycled, another source of pollution that could be regulated, but isn't, as the EPA has yet to set standards for removing the switches from auto scrap. The agency did institute a National Vehicle Mercury Switch Reduction Program to collect and recycle the toxic scrap metal, but exhausted its voluntary incentive fund for the program in 2009.[29]

The state of Texas is home to five of the top ten mercury emitting power plants. The largest such plant in the nation, Luminant's Martin Lake power plant in Dallas, released 1,764 pounds of mercury in 2008, a 4.56 percent increase over the previous year. The plant was the subject of a September 2010 federal lawsuit filed by a coalition of environmental groups led by the Sierra Club for amassing more than 50,000 air pollution violations over its history. Martin Lake power plant is single-handedly responsible for 13 percent of all industrial air pollution in Texas.[30] And Texas' statewide mercury emissions—reported at 11,722 pounds for 2008—dwarf those of other states. Total US mercury emissions for all states combined for that year were 89,422 pounds.[31] The aforementioned 2005 Texas study found a direct relationship between how close families live to areas high in mercury-containing emissions and the likelihood of children being diagnosed with autism and needing special education services. The study looked at mercury totals reported for 2001 in 254 Texas counties—districts that ranged from urban to rural and encompassed some 4 million children. Coal-fired power plants were the largest mercury emitters, followed by medical waste incinerators and commercial boilers. For every 1,000 pounds of environmentally released mercury, there was a 61 percent increase in autism rates. It was the first study to link low-dose exposure to mercury emissions to a developmental disorder, and while causation could not be proved, the study did point to an unsettling link.[32]

Jeff Sell, a former Texas trial lawyer who's now the vice president of public policy at the Autism Society, a leading grassroots autism group, raised his family in Spring, Texas. The town is located just north of Houston in an area known as "Cancer Alley," a 300-mile stretch where Texas and Louisiana meet along the Gulf of Mexico that boasts the largest collection of oil refineries and factories in the world. An Energy Information Administration (EIA) map of Texas shows clusters of triangles so dense they overlap—orange for natural gas plants, black for coal. A collection of "Quick Facts" about the state running alongside the map notes that "Texas' 27 petroleum refineries can process more than 4.7 million barrels of crude oil per day, and they account for more than one-fourth of total US refining capacity."[33]

Sell didn't need a map to know those oil refineries were there. He walked outside his house every day to air thick with the wavy aftereffects. He could smell the sickly benzene on his two boys after they'd been out playing on the backyard swing set. "They smelled like little walking benzene dolls," he says. "They're outside playing for a half hour on the swing set and they come back in and they smell like a damn refinery."[34]

Benzene can pass from a mother's blood to a developing fetus.[35] High levels of exposure can cause drowsiness, dizziness, and tremors. It can also cause leukemia and a decrease in red blood cells. Both of Sell's sons—fraternal twins who are now sixteen years old—have autism. Their autism manifests very differently. Ben is completely nonverbal, still in Pull-Ups with severe behavioral issues. Joe, on the other hand, talks incessantly—not unlike Dustin Hoffman's character in *Rain Man*, according to his dad. While Joe's not good at interacting with peers, Sell says, "he's a big lovable bear who will talk your ear off." Sell's two daughters, eighteen-year-old Natalie, and thirteen-year-old Gracie, are unaffected.

Sell couldn't help but wonder how the toxins surrounding his home might have contributed to his sons' autism, and, in turn, his own health. So he signed on as a participant in a biomonitoring project called "Mind, Disrupted," in which twelve leaders and self advocates from the learning and developmental disability community, as well as one athlete—NFL player David Irons—volunteered to have their blood and urine tested for toxin levels. The participants were tested for eighty-nine substances with known or suspected links to neurodevelopmental disorders. A total of sixty-one chemicals were found in the twelve people tested; each person had at least twenty-six of the chemicals in his or her body, and one had thirty-eight.[36] At nearly 3 ppb, Sell's blood mercury level was well above the CDC average of about 1 part per billion, and the third highest in the study; a mercury level of 5 ppb or more would prompt a necessary medical visit. Another participant, Dr. Robert Fletcher, the founder and CEO of the National Association for the Dually Diagnosed (NADD), which specializes in those with both mental illness and intellectual disabilities, had the fourth-highest mercury levels. He also suffers from dyslexia. "When I was a child, I used to play with mercury quite often," Dr. Fletcher remarked. "My father was a dentist and worked out of the house. Also, years ago, I wasn't aware of any health effects of lead, so I used to bite on the lead weight when I went fishing."[37] Now he wonders if those early exposures contributed to his learning disability—and to the more severe mental impairments he sees every day in his practice.

Sell might have been more focused on his own lingering mercury impacts had he not been so stunned by the level of triclosan in his body,[38] a chemical used to boost the antibacterial and antifungal properties of products from toothpaste to soap, to socks, furniture, and kitchenware. Blood tests revealed Sell had more than 500 parts per million of triclosan coursing through his veins—a level that puts him at about the one hundredth percentile when compared to national averages, and leagues above that of any other participants. Triclosan is an endocrine-disrupting chemical, meaning that even a small dose can potentially wreak havoc on the endocrine system, which regulates everything from mood to growth to metabolism to sexual function. Dr. Irva Hertz-Picciotto, a professor of public health sciences at University of California, Davis who has researched the connection between autism and toxins, says, "We are learning that hormones, such as the sex steroids estrogen and androgen and the thyroxine system and corticosteroids . . . are all essential for proper brain development. In other words, the fetus in utero really responds to how much of these chemicals are circulating and mostly they come from the mother." Antimicrobial chemicals such as triclosan, she says, "seem to be capable of enhancing estrogenic activity. That means that they could potentially play a role in autism or other neurodevelopmental disorders."[39]

Sell's family uses organic bath products and natural cleaners, actively avoiding chemicals and additives. Sell had never even heard of triclosan before they discovered such high levels of it in his body. Since the study, he's tried to reduce his levels, but he remains frustrated. "It's obviously not something I'm doing," Sell says. "It's the microban in my refrigerator, it's that 'new car' smell, clothes are treated with it. I'm a very seasoned individual when it comes to 'going green' and avoiding toxic chemicals, and I felt really stupid. I had no idea what it was, and no idea how to reduce my level of exposure." And Sell is not alone. With the rise in antibacterial products has come a rapid increase in the amount of triclosan turning up in people's bodies after it is absorbed from cosmetics or hand soaps, or ingested during tooth-brushing. In the CDC's most recent public health report, covering 2003–2004, triclosan was found in the urine of nearly 75 percent of the people tested.[40]

It isn't clear whether Sell's triclosan level—or concurrent levels in his wife, who was not studied but surely similarly exposed—could have passed to their boys and altered their development. But it is certain that endocrine disruptors can easily pass from mother to fetus and vastly alter development by changing the way genes are programmed in a baby's developing tissues in utero. The devastating health effects, in some cases, don't arise until during or after puberty. That lesson was learned between the 1950s and 1970s when women were routinely given a synthetic hormone called diethylstilbestrol (DES) as both a "morning after" pill and to combat morning sickness during pregnancy. Daughters born to these mothers were left with a terrible legacy that included a rare, vaginal cancer, reproductive abnormalities, infertility, and miscarriages.[41] While the FDA subsequently withdrew approval for the use of DES in pregnant women, other hormone-mimicking chemicals found in pesticides, cleaners, tainted food, and cosmetics remain in wide production. Hormone-disrupting chemicals are thought to be partially responsible for a host of health disorders as varied as infertility, diabetes, thyroid disorders, ADHD, and autism. The Endocrine Disruption Exchange (TEDX), an organization founded by Dr. Theo Colburn whose sole focus is the impact of low doses of these chemicals, relates on its website that "The endocrine system is so fine tuned that it depends upon changes in hormones in concentrations as little as a tenth of a trillion of a gram to control the womb environment. That's as inconspicuous as one second in 3,169 centuries."[42]

PCBs and the flame retardants known as PBDEs are also hormone-mimicking chemicals that confuse the body's processes by acting as "keys" to the body's pre-programmed "locks." The uterus, for example, doesn't know the difference between estrogen or estrogen-like chemicals. Both real hormones and chemical imitators will initiate certain processes—from regulating ovulation to terminating pregnancy. Once the lock has been fit by an imposter key, the natural key is shut out. The body's thyroid hormones, for example, may be permanently disrupted by the presence of PCBs or other endocrine disruptors in the bloodstream, which flow to their cellular targets and throw off the body's natural system of regulation. When endocrine disruptors like flame retardants get into a developing fetus' bloodstream by way of a pregnant mother eating contaminated fish, eating high amounts of meat and dairy, breathing air near a contaminated site, or inhaling PBDE-laced household dust, they alter the fetus' tissue development and put the fetus at risk of developing a disorder. Research published in the journal *Environmental Health Perspectives* linked exposure to PBDEs with lowered levels of the thyroid-stimulating hormones known as T3 and T4, resulting in hyperthyroidism. When pregnant mothers suffer from hyperthyroidism, their infants' brain development is at significant risk for impairment.[43] A study from the Netherlands found that mothers whose T4 levels were in the lowest tenth percentile of the population during the first trimester of pregnancy were much more likely to give birth to a child with a low IQ or even mild retardation.[44]

PBDEs are chemicals of serious concern in relation to rising autism rates, says Dr. Hertz-Picciotto, despite the fact that many of them are now banned from use and manufacture. "Because they are persistent in the environment, the human body, or both," she says, "they will hang around for a long time, similar to PCBs which were banned decades ago."[45] The EPA concurs, stating, "There is growing evidence that PBDEs persist in the environment and accumulate in living organisms, as well as toxicological testing that indicates these chemicals may cause liver toxicity, thyroid toxicity, and neurodevelopmental toxicity. Environmental monitoring programs in Europe, Asia, North America, and the Arctic have found traces of several PBDEs in human breast milk, fish, aquatic birds, and elsewhere in the environment."[46] The most recent national study from the Centers for Disease Control and Prevention found that nearly everyone had one type of PBDE in their blood; four other related flame retardants were found in more than 60 percent of those studied.[47]

Flame retardants are added to products from Superman pajamas to flooring to computers and TVs. Since flame retardants aren't chemically bound, they can be released in the course of everyday life, accumulating in the environment, in animals, and in people. Sometimes, PBDEs are released by burning; such was the case on September 11, 2001, when al-Qaeda terrorists flew passenger jets into the World Trade Center's Twin Towers in New York City, toppling the buildings, killing 2,752 people, and sending thick plumes of smoke, including toxic dust and fumes, into the surrounding community. Flame retardants were among the many chemicals released en masse from the burning remains. Three months after the attack, the National Institute of Environmental Health Sciences (NIEHS) set out to discover precisely what impact the increased flame retardants from the burning and debris had on babies born nearby. Researchers studied more than 200 cord blood samples taken from mothers who were pregnant on that terrible day and delivered at one of three hospitals located two miles from the World Trade Center site. They tested the children for developmental and neurological delays periodically up through age six. They found that women who delivered their babies the closest to the date of the attacks had the highest cord blood concentrations of PBDEs, and "Children who were in the highest 20 percent of cord blood concentrations of PBDEs... had significantly lower developmental scores compared to children who were in the lower 80 percent," the report noted.[48]

That study was only the second public health study to look at the physical and mental impacts of flame retardants on the prenatal environment, but other studies have indicated the dangers of flame retardants building up in the bloodstreams of developing children. We know that these flame retardants have increased over the years and are present in household dust and released through vacuuming. Flame retardants tend to settle in fats, whether fatty fish and shellfish or high-fat breast milk—and more flame retardants in household dust means more is present in mothers' breast milk. Swedish studies discovered that flame retardants in breast milk had doubled every five years between 1972 and 1997 in that country,[49] and two decades ago government agencies and companies began phasing out PBDEs as a result. The impact was unmistakable: the amount of PBDEs in Swedish women's breast milk fell by nearly 30 percent between 1997 and 2000, from a one-time high of 4 parts per billion of milk fat to 2.79ppb.[50] Most other European countries have followed Sweden's lead in banning PBDEs, as have Canada and a handful of US states.

Because Sweden is the only country that regularly monitors breast milk for chemical intruders, it has been difficult to make meaningful comparisons. But the few studies that have looked at the chemical's concentration in the blood and breast milk of women in the US reveal incredible amounts of PBDEs in our bodies at levels known to cause adverse impacts in animals. In 2003, a group of researchers from Texas analyzed breast milk samples from forty-seven nursing mothers in the state. They found shockingly high concentrations of PBDEs—from 6.2 to 419ppb, with an average level of 73.9ppb. The levels of flame retardants they found mirrored findings in blood and tissue samples from California and Indiana, and, the researchers wrote, "are 10–100 times greater than human tissue levels in Europe." It's quite possible, they conclude, that such PBDE-laced breast milk poses "potential toxicity to nursing infants."[51]

Doctors treating children with autism have seen evidence of thyroid dysfunction that they suspect may be the result of multiple chemical exposures, and it has proven challenging, or even impossible, to treat. Dr. Suruchi Chandra of the True Health Medical Center in Naperville, Illinois, says many of the children with autism she treats have abnormal thyroid tests, but treating their thyroid problems is complicated by the fact that the test results don't fit any classic assessment such as hyperthyroidism. "When I see these abnormalities I usually refer these children to the pediatric endocrinologist for further evaluation and treatment, especially because we know how involved the thyroid gland is in brain development in childhood," she says. "Usually the assessment I get back from the pediatric endocrinologist is 'unspecified abnormal thyroid test results.' So they're not sure how to interpret these test results and no treatment is offered because the test results don't fit any conventional diagnostic categories. And my concern and hypothesis is that in part these abnormal thyroid function tests are due to the numerous common and widespread chemicals that are known to be thyroid hormone disruptors. . . . PCBs, dioxins, certain flame retardants, phthalates and BPA . . . it's impossible for a child to go throughout the day and not be exposed to one of these chemicals and most likely many of these chemicals."[52]

Thyroid problems are not the only bodily disruption likely connected to a chemical that Dr. Chandra sees in children with autism. Many of her patients also suffer from mitochondrial and immune dysfunction. In the case of the former, the mitochondria—or "powerhouses" of the cell—are not functioning properly, a condition that Dr. Chandra says can lead to "developmental and growth delays, low muscle tone, chronic constipation, and a host of other symptoms." The body's immune system is just as crucial for proper development; it protects the body from disease and infection and is necessary to prevent against a host of brain disorders, including autism. "These biomedical conditions that we often see in children are multifactorial in origin," she says. "It's not as simple as saying they're caused by environmental toxins. There are a number of factors, and they usually include genetic vulnerability, poor nutrition, stress, drugs, and exposure to environmental toxins." Increasingly problematic in all these cases, she adds, is that doctors are not trained to recognize and treat conditions that arise from chemical exposures, and the persistent difficulty in assessing such exposures in the first place. "We don't have much training in the impact of environmental toxins," Dr. Chandra says. "I had no training during my medical school or residency. And also there's no simple way of measuring the type of toxicity we're referring to. It's not one substance that the child's ingesting at one time that you can simply measure with a blood test. We're talking about prolonged exposure over years to many toxins. And there's no simple way of quantitatively measuring that type of toxicity."[53]

Should we stop eating fish? Stop nursing babies? Stop having babies? Should we all move to Washington, Maine, Oregon, Vermont, Rhode Island, Illinois or Massachusetts—the few states that have banned all or some highly toxic PBDEs? These are the ludicrous questions parents-to-be must now ask until Congress passes decisive regulation protecting human health. Laura Abulafia, the director of the Environmental Health Initiative at the American Association on Intellectual and Developmental Disabilities in California, and one of the Mind, Disrupted participants, had blood mercury levels higher than anyone else in the study—nearly 8 parts per billion—one of only two whose mercury levels registered above the 95th percentile. Abulafia was recently married and wants to have kids some day, but she's scared of the toxic burden she can't help but pass along. "I'm deeply disturbed and feel very helpless that these known toxic chemicals are still being used, still left unregulated," the young woman says. "Should my child be born with a serious disability or disorder, it would be a terrible responsibility wondering what I did wrong or what I could have done differently. I don't want to live in fear that the food I eat and the products I use will impact my future children. And I shouldn't have to. None of us should have to."[54]

THREE

Dumped On
When Chemicals Act in Combination

There's nothing remarkable about French's Landfill today. Without the fence and the "Danger" signs, this Superfund site—a designation for the most complex abandoned hazardous waste sites—tucked into a residential community between the Garden State Parkway and a local high school in Brick Township, New Jersey, is just another overgrown remnant from the past. Nature has largely taken over the former dump's forty-two acres. Now, trees spread their canopies and animals build their nests. But from 1949 until its closing in 1979, the dump held the waste of the area's factories, industries, stores, and homes—the garbage, construction debris, vegetable and sewage wastes; the engine oil, anti-freeze, resin, pesticides, and herbicides.[1] Between 1969 and 1979, the New Jersey Department of Environmental Protection (NJDEP) and the EPA estimate that 63 million gallons of septic waste were collected at French's.[2]

Only later were the impacts of all that waste assessed. Heavy metals and volatile organic compounds (VOCs) had leaked out of their storage containers, tainting the soil and local groundwater supplies. There were twenty-four worrisome contaminants in all, including benzene (used to make plastics, dyes, and detergents), chloroform (the one-time anesthetic, now used to make other chemicals), tetrachloroethylene (used in dry cleaning and degreasing metals), vinyl chloride, pesticides, ammonia, and metals, including arsenic, cadmium, mercury, and nickel. In 1982, the town removed the drums, and in 1983, the landfill was placed on the EPA's Superfund National Priorities List. But the damage was done. In the late 1990s, after years of officials battling over whether to install an impermeable cap with a methane gas ventilation system over the site, an operation that would have cost the town $10 million it didn't want to spend, they discovered that the chemicals had already escaped their fenced-in perimeter and migrated in a "kidney-shaped" plume into residents' groundwater. In 1999 the town was forced to ban the use of groundwater in a one-mile perimeter of the landfill. Residents were shifted to a municipal water supply, and in 2001, local officials sealed 270 contaminated area wells.[3]

Bobbie and Billy Gallagher and their three children live just a few streets away from the abandoned landfill on Carroll Fox Road, a desirable part of the seaside town where older homes with years of lived-in and added-on character are each fronted by pretty patches of yard. The Gallaghers's home is a weathered white Cape Cod built in the 1930s. The original owner was a builder who added rooms as his budget allowed, so the house meanders in shape: a sun porch tacked on one side, a laundry room on another.

The home's décor has gone in a distinctly Disney direction. On the living room mantle is an elaborate *Little Mermaid*-themed scene, including silver netting, an Ariel doll perched on a shell, a treasure chest, and a hanging stuffed clownfish that Bobbie had originally set up around Christmas. Nearly a year later, the scene remains because her two profoundly autistic children, Alana, age nineteen, and Austin, age eighteen, are Disney fanatics who can't bear to see it go. Under a clear plastic cover on the dining room table, completed puzzles feature scenes from more Disney movies: *Lady and the Tramp*, *Sleeping Beauty*, and *Finding Nemo*. Even their oversized dog is named Bruno, after the dog in Cinderella. The Gallaghers's oldest child, Chelsea, does not have autism; she is a twenty-one-year-old student at Stockton College in Ponoma, New Jersey, who was awarded "hero of the year" at her school for a campaign she organized against teenage drunk driving. "I always tease that she's the one that proves that I could have done this right if I had three typical kids," Bobbie says. "I at least know that I was on the right track of being a good mom because Chelsea came out to be such a good kid."

Though her two children with autism have reached adult age physically, they are in many respects like overgrown toddlers who lack the language skills that help children begin to navigate their worlds with a degree of independence. They get their demands met by repeating phrases, noises, and frustrated whines; they are aloof and needy simultaneously, trapped inside their own worlds, where each daily task or event must adhere to a specific, individual order. Alana, who has a shock of short, bright red hair and pale skin, is friendly, interested in people, and the more verbal of the two. She's a "scriptor," who quotes from Disney movies at random, sometimes even applying a line that fits the situation at hand. If her mother asks, "Alana, where are you going?," she might reply, "Promise or no promise, I can't stay here another minute!"—a line from *Beauty and the Beast*. Alana's memory is full of details—particularly dates—and she is obsessed with knowing the coming events for the days ahead, no matter how mundane. That can lead to problems when a planned activity doesn't come to pass because dad is stuck in traffic, the car breaks down, or the power goes out. On these occasions, she will stand behind her mother and remind relentlessly. If her calendar says she is supposed to go to McDonald's at 5:00, and life intervenes, Bobbie says, "She won't leave you alone. She'll stand behind you and say 'Mommy, McDonald's, 5:00. It's 5:02.'"[4] As the minutes tick by, she keeps reminding, becoming increasingly agitated as the promised trip does not materialize at its designated time. Alana craves structure and lists, and will gladly perform chores—taking out the garbage, doing the laundry, and cleaning her room—but any free time makes her anxious.

Austin is Alana's opposite in many respects. He still has a baby face, and speaks and interacts far less than his sister. Austin is content to stay in his room all day and watch videos, and he needs powerful motivations to complete even simple tasks. For him to agree to take a bath—which he does every other day—he wants french fries or chips in exchange. His fisherman father's love for the water has manifested in Austin; he can amuse himself for long stretches standing in an inflatable pool in the back yard, sending streams of water straight up into the air with a cupped hand, a trick no one in the family has yet been able to imitate. A piercing alarm is activated inside the house if he attempts to leave the backyard perimeter. Both Austin and Alana love parasailing, but it is Austin whose face turns to sheer joy when he is bobbing above the waves from the back of a boat. He has always craved heights, his mother says, and as a young child would often climb on top of the mantle when her back was turned, or to the very top of a playscape, like the king of his own private kingdom. As he has grown older, Austin has been challenging in ways that Alana has not. His frustration can quickly turn to aggression; he's capable of injuring himself or others. Neither child can ever be left alone.

Because her two children with autism are so close in age—just fourteen months apart—Bobbie learned about their autism in quick succession. When Alana was eighteen months old and still not saying "Mama" or responding to her name, friends and family told her not to worry, and not to compare her to Chelsea, who had been an early talker and could name colors like "lavender" and "turquoise" at the same age. A visit with an audiologist confirmed that Alana could definitely hear sounds; a follow-up visit with a speech therapist made it official that

Alana had autism. By then Alana had become a toddler, and her parents began noticing certain peculiarities with the new baby, Austin. He made eye contact and smiled, but he never responded to sounds. When Bobbie banged pots and pans behind Austin he didn't budge or react. They suspected their youngest son was deaf. Bobbie took him to have his hearing tested, sitting in a booth with her baby as they exposed him to lights and sounds, watching for a reaction that never came. They concluded Austin was deaf, and Bobbie took the news in stride. She remembers thinking, "OK, I can handle deaf. I can learn sign language." In many ways, a diagnosis of deaf seemed safer—more predictable—than another autism diagnosis.

But at a follow-up visit to a neurologist, Austin was given the brainstem auditory evoked response, or BAER, test. They put electrodes on his head and headphones over his ears, and administered sounds to see if those sounds were registering in his brain. They were. The doctor told Bobbie, "He can hear. I'm not sure what the problem is, but it's not the ears." Bobbie knew immediately that Austin, too, had autism. "I made an appointment with the neurologist for Austin, just to get the autism diagnosis so I could get the services he needed," Bobbie says. "But I already knew."

Those early days were so challenging, the parents could focus on little else but soldiering through. Where most babies have a variety of cries that parents learn to decipher—a whimper that means "I'm sleepy," a discomfort cry that means "I need a diaper change," and a wail that translates as "I'm hurt"—Alana and Austin both had what Bobbie calls "one ear-piercing, hair-raising screech." She had to eliminate possibilities one by one every time either one of them cried. "It was always as if the world was about to come to an end each and every time," Bobbie says.

It was only after Alana turned three and was in a special school that Bobbie reached out to a local autism support group, Families for Autistic Children Education and Support (FACES), run by Autism New Jersey. She quickly noticed something unusual about the new moms who came to weekly meetings: all of them were from Brick Township, and all had children around the same age. At a workshop run by the organization a presenter approached Bobbie and asked, "What's going on in your town?" The presenter said she'd been receiving multiple calls each week from families looking for support services, and all of them lived in Brick. Bobbie began suspecting that there was an autism cluster in her area; was the autism that had touched her family twice not merely a construct of fate and genetics, but triggered by something else in their immediate environment? Her first thought was that it might be something in the water.

French's Landfill, which had seeped contaminants into Brick's soil and wells, had forced the town to shift residents to drinking water drawn from the Metedeconk River, a favorite place for boating, fishing, paddling, and swimming. Unlike groundwater, surface water (in other words, water drawn from the river) needs more treatment before it is considered drinkable; surface water doesn't have the benefit of filtering through the grainy soil. The water treatment plant that filtered Metedoconk River water is located one street behind the Gallaghers's home.

Bobbie's concerns about her family's water supply came straight from her own bathtub. Sometimes when she filled it the water looked blue against the white tub. It wasn't until Alana and Austin were well into their toddler years that she learned that drinking contaminated water is not necessarily the most likely path of toxin exposure; hot baths and showers, particularly very hot, very steamy ones, can result in breathing contaminants from the water directly into the lungs, or absorbing water through the skin's enlarged pores. Like most moms, Bobbie knew she wasn't supposed to eat too many tuna fish sandwiches or smoke cigarettes while pregnant, but no one had ever said "be careful how hot your showers are." Bobbie admits she favors a shower that is practically scalding, one that leaves her skin pink, even in the summer. One study found that blood levels of trichloroethylene (TCE), a toxic solvent used for degreasing metal (exposure to which has been found to cause a marked increase in one's likelihood of developing Parkinson's Disease[5]), were highest in people who had showered for ten minutes, intermediate for those who bathed for ten minutes, and lowest for those who drank a liter of water, all from the same water source.[6]

Before anyone would test the water, Bobbie needed an official determination that there was an actual autism cluster. That process exposed her to a world of bureaucratic, political, and legal wrangling that seemed designed to wear her down. She started by contacting area families the only way she knew how: she composed a simple survey that asked if families had a child with autism, and whether that child was born in Brick. The public school refused to distribute the survey, so Bobbie left it in library bins, handed it out to area parents, and e-mailed it to other locals. The survey was designed to weed out any families who had simply moved to Brick to take advantage of the town's autism services. More than forty people responded and fit the criteria. Convinced they indeed had a cluster, Bobbie partnered with the National Alliance for Autism Research (a group that has since been absorbed into the larger Autism Speaks) for a meeting and strategy session at the local library, with about seventy in attendance.

At the time, in the late 1990s, autism clusters were unheard of. Researchers in the US had only just begun to study autism's rising numbers at the time Bobbie was becoming concerned about a possible cluster in her community. The largest comprehensive look at autism prevalence then underway was taking place in metropolitan Atlanta; the results of research there led the CDC to estimate that 3.4 of every 1,000 children had some form of autism, with a male-to-female ratio of 4:1. That didn't offer Bobbie much as a basis for comparison, other than to make it clear that autism rates were increasing, with rates ten times higher than previous measurements from the 1980s and early 1990s.[7]

Autism had yet to gain status as a Major Public Concern, complete with the requisite magnetic car ribbons. It wasn't yet drawing the research dollars of health concerns like cancer. Just a few years prior to Bobbie's launching her investigation into autism cases in her community, nearby Tom's River, New Jersey, had been identified as having a childhood cancer cluster—one that panicked residents felt sure was due to the town's two Superfund sites that were contaminating area air and water. The issue garnered plenty of media publicity, public support, and $1 million in Congressional funding to launch a federal investigation. The results of the study, in the end, were deemed inconclusive, in that officials could not link the cancer and leukemia rates with a specific contaminant, but they did find that moms exposed to airborne emissions from the Ciba-Geigy plant, a dye and chemical factory, were more likely to give birth to daughters with leukemia.[8] Preempting any potential lawsuits, in 2002 the companies responsible for the toxins—Union Carbide, Ciba Specialty Chemicals, and United Water Toms River—agreed to a multimillion dollar settlement with sixty-nine families who had children with cancer, without ever admitting liability. Residents of 700 homes who pursued a class-action suit were awarded a $20 million settlement from Ciba-Geigy in June 2011.[9]

Bobbie wasn't likely to obtain the same sort of public attention or outrage as the residents of Tom's River (as one official told her, "Cancer is sexy"), but the nearby cancer cluster loomed large in everyone's minds—and that made local politicians, in particular, very uneasy. At the time, Brick's mayor was Joseph C. Scarpelli, a politician who would later serve an eighteen-month federal prison sentence for accepting bribes. When Bobbie and Billy told the mayor that they thought the autism rates in Brick deserved a thorough investigation, he responded, "Let's not turn this into another Tom's River, OK?"

"The only thing I was looking for—and I was hoping the other parents would want [this]—was [for] the children . . . born in Brick Township . . . [to] be able to live in Brick Township for the rest of their lives with their families and have other outlets as they grew older," Bobbie says. "We should start developing some programs for them so they'll have full lives. I'm not bitter about having children with autism.

I'm perfectly fine with raising them until I can no longer walk—but I wanted to have places where I could take them and do things with them and feel like I was in a community of people who were accepting of us."

When the CDC finally began to examine data to determine the prevalence of autism in Brick, a local attorney's office took out a full-page newspaper ad in search of families ready to sue. Representatives from the CDC argued over whether to call the autism rates "elevated" in their final report, making it seem to Bobbie as though word choice was more important to officials than discovering what was wrong. The ATSDR, tasked with determining the levels of chemicals in residents' drinking water during the time period in question, relied on the water company's own data; no independent sampling of the air and water in residents' household dust, or of the blood and urine of affected family members, was done.

After completing the studies, officials from the CDC and ATSDR merely called everyone back to the local library and passed out two long documents, one from each agency, detailing the results. The officials said people were welcome to take a seat and read the results, and if they had any questions, they would be waiting to answer them. The CDC's final report in 1998 concluded that there were "high rates of autistic disorder and ASD in Brick Township relative to rates from previously published studies." But because the sample population was so small, and because there was so little data on autism prevalence available for the rest of the country, they could not interpret those numbers as having any statistical meaning. The ATSDR, which had looked at the chemical concentrations in the local drinking water, did find levels of THM exceeding the EPA's maximum allowed contaminant level of eighty parts per billion, but they couldn't link these higher concentrations to the autism cases in question, writing that "the locations in the water system where total THM levels were high do not match the locations and timing of the pregnancies of the majority of the autism cases plotted." They concluded it was unlikely that THM was a factor in Brick's higher autism numbers.[10]

Without independent testing, or any testing at all of the participants or their homes, Bobbie found these conclusions hard to accept. But the frustrating process of investigating the issue had begun to wear on her, and her neighbors had grown wary of the public attention her efforts were generating. They had their property values to consider, after all. The Gallaghers and other families who prompted the investigation began to doubt that anyone was really looking to find answers. It was beginning to seem as though this quest was all about money—how much money could be secured for the investigation; how much money lawyers thought they could sue for; how much money homes were worth now and would be later; how much money local officials were willing to spend to cap the dump that was leaking chemicals.

The answer to that last question could be answered: they would spend as little as they had to. Bobbie recalls how Mayor Scarpelli bragged at the time that he'd saved the town millions of dollars by not implementing the impermeable concrete cap for French's Landfill as had been recommended. Instead, the agency charged with protecting the state's environment reversed its own findings and determined that such a cap would not be necessary and could be replaced instead with a sandy fill, fencing, and groundwater monitoring. Since two feet of sandy fill had already been put on the site in 1979, they had nothing left to do but add a fence and check the water. The fence was put in, but after 1991, the water testing stopped. When the NJDEP resumed water monitoring in 1997, the agency found that toxic compounds remained in the groundwater. In fact, since those wells touched by the toxic plume were sealed, the toxins remained, and some concentrations were even on the rise, according to one EPA report. As of 2007, groundwater still contained higher-than-recommended concentrations of vinyl chloride, benzene, arsenic, and mercury,[11] and political wrangling over how to finally clean up the contaminated dump continues, more than thirty years after the landfill was officially closed.

At the same time that the Brick investigation was winding its way to its inconclusive end, an investigative report called "Inconclusive By Design: Waste, Fraud, and Abuse in Federal Environmental Health Research" was released. The report was published by the Environmental Health Network, a California-based consumer advocacy group alerting people to common health dangers in their environment, as well as the National Toxics Campaign Fund, one of the few national groups fighting toxins in the US from the mid-eighties to early nineties (the group closed in 1993). It takes to task the very agencies—the CDC and the ATSDR—that were responsible for finding answers for the elevated autism numbers in Brick.

During the course of the federal investigation into Brick Township's water supply, a member of Physicians for Social Responsibility handed Bobbie Gallagher a copy of the "Inconclusive By Design" report. Its lessons would stay with her. The CDC's focus on word choice instead of causes, the lack of testing of families or homes, the impersonal wrap-up when the investigation ended—it all seemed orchestrated to pacify the public, to push the whole messy business out of sight until the upset died down.

Despite scientific evidence that chemicals from hazardous waste sites can cause direct health problems ranging from cancer to birth defects, "Inconclusive By Design" charges that the agencies responsible for investigating these toxins and protecting the public health are more often soothing ruffled feathers instead. The CDC and ATSDR have become "virtual propaganda tools of polluting industries," the report finds, "making public reassurance instead of public protection their foremost focus. One result has been an increase in public complacency and government inaction at many sites where further precautions to reduce toxic exposures are necessary." The report finds inherent problems with the way such investigations were carried out, like using statistical studies on small, mobile populations and refusing to fully engage with the people being studied. Statistics don't work on small populations; even if autism rates, in the case of Brick, were "double or triple the normal rate for the population, in many small communities this would not be high enough for statisticians to confirm the link between exposure and disease." Thus, the use of statistics to measure these populations almost always leads to an "inconclusive" diagnosis.

In the case of CDC studies of Superfund sites and public health problems, the groups found that the CDC failed to adequately involve affected residents. In Jacksonville, Arkansas, for example, where the Vietnam-era herbicide Agent Orange was manufactured, there was a spike in cases of sudden infant death syndrome (SIDS) surrounding an area where the chemicals had been dumped. But the CDC "refused to test the tissues of one hundred SIDS victims which a physician at the Arkansas Children's Hospital believed to contain high levels of toxic chemicals." ATSDR, meanwhile, was criticized for failing to interact with local populations or to inform them when toxic health assessments had been made.[12]

At the time the report was published, one-sixth of Americans lived within four miles of a chemical dump or hazardous waste site. More recent estimates by the ATSDR find that one in four Americans now live within four miles of a hazardous waste site.[13] Study after study has indicated that children born to mothers living in close proximity to such toxic sites have an increased risk (12–17 percent, in one study) of being born with abnormalities, including physical birth defects, malformations of the heart and circulatory system, low birth weights, and neural tube defects[14]—the latter two of which can act as precursors to autism. In general, a neural tube defect refers to any disorder involving incomplete formation of the brain, spinal cord, or the surrounding nerves and protective coverings. The most common such disorder is spina bifida, which is when the fetus' spine fails to close properly during the first month of pregnancy, leaving an infant with some amount of paralysis from the waist down. Since 1992, when doctors began recommending that expectant mothers take daily folic acid supplements, incidents of spina bifida and other neural tube defects have fallen dramatically. Thanks to folic acid supplements, spina bifada rates fell by 25 percent from 1995 to 2000 and another 13 percent from 2000 to 2005.[15] As of 2005 there were just 18 cases of spina bifada and anencephaly (another neural tube defect) per 100,000 births in the US.[16] However, a study published in 1994 discovered that an injury occurring at the time the brain and spinal cord (or neural tube) is closing in a developing fetus can lead to autism, too.[17] It was found that thalidomide (a sedative administered to women in the late 1950s and early 1960s to combat morning sickness that resulted in 10,000 children around the world being born with severe birth defects[18]), is a powerful teratogen, a type of drug that also causes malformations in children's eyes, ears, hearts, genitals, kidneys, digestive tracts, and nervous systems. When introduced during a very particular point of development, specifically between the twentieth and twenty-fourth day of gestation, the time period when the neural tube closes (and before many women even know they are pregnant), thalidomide could also cause autism. Valproic acid, a medication used to treat seizures, was also found to cause autism when introduced in rats at the time of neural tube closure.[19] The physical signs that accompanied these drug-induced autism cases included ears that were under-formed or folded over and low-set, along with hearing problems. Victims also experienced paralysis of both the face and eye muscles. "The cranio-facial symptoms have been ignored in the autism literature, because they seem trivial in comparison to the disabling behavioral symptoms," reports Patricia Rodier in her study "Role of Developmental Neurotoxicology in Autism," "but they speak directly to the embryological origin of the disorder."[20]

The ATSDR found three pollutants in Brick's drinking water that exceeded acceptable levels: bromoform, chloroform, and tetrachloroethylene. Bromoform and chloroform are THMs, byproducts of disinfecting the water with chlorine that cause an increased risk for neural tube defects in babies when pregnant mothers are exposed. Tetrachloroethylene (also known as perchlorethylene, or PCE), a chemical used in dry cleaning and metal degreasing, has also been linked to neural tube defects. In its public health assessment following the Brick investigation, the agency acknowledged that these pollutants have been definitively linked to higher rates of neural tube defects, and that introducing certain chemicals between the twentieth and twenty-fourth days of fetal development could cause autism. The agency reported, "This evidence suggests [an] hypothesis that the period when the neural tube closes may also be a period when exposures to certain chemicals might lead to the development of an ASD. It also suggests an hypothesis that chemicals that cause NTD [neural tube defects], since they act during this period of gestation, might also cause ASD. However, research on these hypotheses is at a very early stage. Therefore, it is currently unknown whether in utero exposure to environmental chemicals such as the disinfection byproducts of chlorination are associated with ASD."[21]

Several years after the Brick autism investigations were filed away with other public health mysteries, a researcher named Carol Reinisch, director of the Laboratory of Aquatic Biomedicine at the Marine Biological Laboratory in Woods Hole, Massachusetts, decided to reopen the case. "I was looking for areas where there might be a link between episodes of some type of disease and aquatic-type pollution," Reinisch says, "and I stumbled on Brick."[22] The ATSDR had determined that the pollutants in Brick's water supply—bromoform, chloroform, and tetrachloroethylene—did not individually increase area children's risk for autism. But Reinisch had a novel idea; perhaps it was not these three pollutants acting independently that might trigger autism in developing fetuses, but the effect of them acting together. She tested her theory on simple subjects: surf clam embryos. These transparent invertebrates have very basic bodily systems, making toxic impacts easy to assess. Ideally, if a researcher finds results with clam embryos, she'll take her study up through the vertebrate chain to more complex organisms like mice and rats, nearing humans with each subsequent step.

Reinisch's theory worked. The three toxins, when introduced independently, did not elicit significant changes in the clam embryos. But when they were administered together, the chemical cocktail produced specific neurological changes. The mixture increased production of part of an enzyme called protein kinase A (PKA), which is involved in how neurons in the brain develop and how neural networks are constructed.[23] It was not enough evidence to determine that the pollutants in Brick's water caused autism, but it made a solid case for the fact that toxins in combination can have a unique impact on the way brains develop. And it mirrored the prevailing wisdom about autism's environmental connection—that it is likely not one bodily insult that's driving up cases, but a number of contaminants and exposures acting in concert. "It's very hard to unravel," says Reinisch. "The fact is, autism is a black box. I'm not a neurologist, but it seems to me the real crux in autism will come down to looking at the epidemiology of distinct diseases related to exactly where mothers live during the pregnancy. That's it. Most of the [brain's neural] networks are laid down during pregnancy."[24]

Jill Kreiling, a molecular biologist at Brown University who worked with Reinisch on the surf clam embryo study, wanted to find out if the results would hold true moving up the organism hierarchy. She chose the zebrafish, a vertebrate, and her preliminary findings mirrored the results of the surf clam study. Despite years of effort, however, Kreiling was never able to get a full study funded through the National Institutes of Health (NIH). Such funding is competitive; according to Kreiling, only 8 to 10 percent of studies presented to the NIH are green-lighted. "We feel there's something there," says Kreiling, "but we need funding to prove it."[25]

Dr. Sara Guariglia took up the challenge in 2010 in her doctoral dissertation for City University of New York, applying the same triple threat toxins, first to zebrafish, then to mice. The autism-like impacts on the subjects were unmistakeable. In the case of zebrafish, the combination of bromoform, chloroform, and tetrachloroethylene increased PKA activity, as it had in clam embryos. In the case of mice exposed to the toxins through their drinking water, the disinfectants caused "an increase in the activity of PKA in the cerebral cortex of male animals" on the fourth and tenth days following birth. The brains of female mice were unaffected. What's more, male mice displayed behaviors specific to autism. "Behaviorally, we found that the THM/PCE exposed males develop autistic-like behavioral pathology as they evidence deficits in communication and social behavior and demonstrate both perseverance behavior and anxiety." The behavior of female mice was unaffected. Dr. Guariglia concludes, "These findings suggest that these chemicals may be involved in the etiology of autism and that males are more susceptible to this set of insults."[26]

There are approximately 1,300 Superfund sites on the National Priorities List across the US[27] containing some combination of toxic contaminants like arsenic and asbestos, cadmium and copper, lead and mercury, PCBs and trichloroethene, and vinyl chloride and zinc. In New Jersey there are more than 200 sites that the EPA has identified as needing cleanup as of 2011, including 144 on the National Priorities List.[28] But when US senators sought to uncover the details regarding human exposure to toxins at these sites, they reported being met with secrecy. "It is really stunning to see the casual way EPA treats the public's right to know," Senator Barbara Boxer told The Center for Public Integrity, which tracks the location and mismanagement of Superfund sites, in 2007. "Many of the documents I have asked for at these sites, especially those relating to timing of cleanup, funding shortfalls, and related tasks are stamped 'PRIVILEGED' across the whole page in bright red ink."[29]

Since the 2008 appointment of Lisa Jackson as EPA administrator under President Obama, the agency has ushered in a new era of increased transparency and public education, but securing funds to fully monitor and clean up the nation's most toxic sites remains a constant challenge. In some cases, the companies responsible for the multimillion dollar cleanup costs declare bankruptcy to avoid the payments, leaving much of the cost to be borne by taxpayers. In other cases, the original polluters have long since disappeared. If no responsible party exists, the "EPA will investigate the full extent of the contamination before starting significant clean up,"[30] the agency attests—but this process can take years. Then the agency must offer possible strategies for dealing with the sites and review remedies that exceed $25 million.[31] Meanwhile, the ATSDR keeps the public informed by publishing toxicological profiles of 310 priority substances that may be part of the contamination stew at any one of these sites. The fact that many toxins on the list are nearly unpronounceable does little to soothe worried minds. The agencies may be doing a better job of providing the public with the facts, but solutions are still hard to come by.

New Jersey had the highest recorded autism rates in the country—1 in 94 as of 2002—but that number has lost some of its impact with the release of 2006 data indicating that one in 83 eight-year-olds in Arizona and Missouri have the disorder and the national average has shifted to 1 in 110 kids.[32] Since the investigation that took place in Brick, families in other parts of the country have discovered unusual numbers of kids with autism in their immediate regions, but the US has yet to officially recognize an autism cluster. The investigation in California that turned out to be a "false alarm"—since the unusually high rate of diagnosed autism cases was found to be related to parental affluence and access to services, rather than any certain pollutant—put the issue of environmental contamination as a major autism driver to rest for some. But just as Bobbie began noticing the rate of autism in her community was far above average when she began attending local autism support groups, occasionally parents become aware that their own struggles with autism are not isolated—that they are surrounded by what seems to be unusually high numbers of other families struggling with autism within mere neighborhood blocks.

That was the case in the small Washington DC suburb of Centreville, Virginia, located in wealthy Fairfax County, home of the Central Intelligence Agency, the National Reconnaissance Office, and the National Counterterrorism Center. In 2009 Centreville mothers became aware that there were at least six boys with autism living within blocks of one another, all of whom had been born and raised there. Seeking answers, one of the mothers was told by the Virginia Health Department that it did not collect data on autism. Nor would the CDC initiate a study, since the state health department had not requested one. When a local news station made inquiries about the possible cluster, the Virginia Department of Mental Health responded, "We have a lot on our plate."[33] There are a host of polluting industries located in Fairfax County: the EPA's Toxic Release Inventory for the county cites BP Products North America releasing 2,822 pounds of toxins per year; the Newington Concrete Plant as releasing 171 pounds of toxins; the Sipca Securink Corporation, which makes security inks for banknotes, releasing 250 pounds of toxins; the Virginia Concrete Edsall Road Plant releasing 154 pounds of toxins; and several petroleum and concrete operations for which pollution data is not available.[34] Concerns were also raised about Dulles International Airport, a potent source of area air pollution in the form of carbon monoxide, nitrogen oxide, and particulate matter—most of it the result of the constant operation of fossil-fuel burning cars, trucks, and transport vehicles on the ground.[35]

Questions also remain over a possible autism cluster in Northvale, New Jersey. In 2007, teachers at St. Anthony's School reported giving birth to children with higher-than-average rates of neurodevelopmental disorders and autism. The parochial school itself had been closed in 1978 as a result of low enrollment, but special education classes for up to eighty-five students with autism and learning disabilities continued in the building until 2007 when teachers raised health concerns. Of the 54 children born to 28 women who had worked at St. Anthony's during a 15-year span, 28 of them, or 52 percent, had a neurodevelopmental disorder, and 10 of these, or 18.5 percent, were diagnosed with an ASD. Nine of the 28 women who met the study criteria worked at St. Anthony's full-time, and had a total of 18 children. Among those, 12 of the 18 children, or 67 percent, had a neurodevelopmental disorder, including 7, or 39 percent, with autism. Nine of the 10 children with autism were boys, and none of their mothers had a family history of autism. A thorough study of the population undertaken by the Deirdre Imus Environmental Center for Pediatric Oncology found that the numbers were significantly higher statistically than those of a control group of children born to teachers at another Northvale public elementary school, and higher than state and national averages. They have yet to connect the higher numbers with any environmental culprit,[36] but several underground storage sites on Walnut Street, where St. Anthony's School is located, have been identified on a list of New Jersey's Known Contaminated Sites, including Flexabar Corporation, which makes industrial coatings for flame-retardant products, primers, gym mats, marine and sports nets, and coatings for life jackets, pool floats, gym mats, and other uses. The company—with yearly sales of some $6.5 million—has been repeatedly fined for violating the EPA's pesticide labeling and distribution regulations, exporting unregistered pesticides abroad, and failing to properly label and identify dangerous pesticides.[37] Also on Walnut Street is the abandoned factory building for Bush Boake Allen Inc., which was bought by International Flavors and Fragrances, then bought again by International Paper. It once housed the makings of chemical flavors and fragrances used in foods, beverages, soaps, detergents, and personal care products.[38] A potent combination of solvents was used to create these chemicals, including the toxic dry cleaning fluid TCE, which has been found in at least 852 of the EPA's approximately 1,300 National Priorities List sites.[39]

The groundwork for uncovering environmental connections to autism has been laid, but tracing possible contamination sources to higher rates of autism within specific communities has proven impossible to date. Even when suspicions are high—where mothers are giving birth to clearly elevated numbers of children with autism—the lack of data, inadequate testing, cost considerations, and political unwillingness to investigate prevent the dots from being connected. Contaminated sites, from chemical storage facilities, to former factory buildings, to toxic landfills, to rail yards and refineries, continue fouling community air, soil, and drinking water, and even serve as building sites for schools or day care centers. The EPA's 2011 voluntary school siting guidelines have been designed to help cities and towns construct new schools that are energy-efficient, maximize walking and biking opportunities, and minimize dangerous environmental exposures.[40] But the guidelines will have little impact on existing schools, particularly urban schools where pristine acreage is hard to come by, and where dangerous levels of exposures are routine, and, in any case, schools will not be required—but only encouraged—to follow them. "Contamination from past industrial activities . . . has been discovered at 11 existing schools in Los Angeles alone during excavation for new classrooms and gymnasiums," reports one article from the Center for Public Environmental Oversight (CPEO); and, according to CPEO, in just California, Massachusetts, Michigan, New Jersey, and New York—"1,100 schools have been built within a half mile of federal or state hazardous waste sites," putting at risk "more than 600,000 children who attend those schools."[41] Once the kids are there, it's a Herculean task for school districts to undertake the remediation measures needed to make a site safe; with so many states across the country buckling under the weight of budget shortfalls, it is not a measure most are willing or able to undertake.

Stephenie Hendricks, a public information director at Pesticide Action Network North America (PANNA) and a mother herself, expresses the frustration many parents feel when faced with a world full of chemical unknowns. "It's random," she says. "There's no way of knowing all the health effects—all the combination of factors including genetics that leads to health problems. Industry would like us to believe that when there's a cluster of health effects that people are too fat, that they smoke too much. Those are the key messaging points—it's the sick person's fault."[42]

For now, parents and doctors must wait for the results of more comprehensive studies of particular communities to determine if there are clusters of autism and to uncover the chemicals and other toxic insults that give rise to those clusters. One such study is the Early Autism Risk Longitudinal Investigation (EARLI), in which researchers plan to follow 1,200 mothers who already have a child with autism through another pregnancy, examining the new child from conception to three years of age and looking for genetic risk factors, environmental exposures, and biological markers that may point to autism. Researchers are studying the mothers' and babies' blood, the placenta, cord blood, the babies' feces, and mothers' breast milk. EARLI has sites in four communities: one in southeast Pennsylvania, one in northeast Maryland, and two in northern California. As of March 2011, EARLI had recruited just 100 families to participate, and had just begun its ten-year quest for answers.[43] There are similar investigations underway across the country.

Broad, nationwide support for such studies is beginning to mount. Many major national autism advocacy organizations are recognizing the importance of environmental research. Autism Speaks, the largest advocacy group, has launched an Environmental Factors in Autism Initiative. If studies prove that contaminants are in fact fueling the increase in autism, families will not be pacified by agency findings that are "inconclusive by design"—even if that means coming to terms with where they live and the potential health hazards in their own back yards. "I was really surprised by the number of people who didn't want it to be the environment because that somehow reflected on their choice of where to live," Bobbie says of her talks with parents of children with autism. "One dad got very upset with us and said, 'I moved out of North Jersey to come down here because it's so good down here,' as if to say: 'You did this.' Most people have no idea that this huge piece of land that says 'Danger' is a Superfund site. A lot of people were like, 'Do you know what you're going to do to the value of my home?' I live here, too, and it never crossed my mind."

FOUR

Gut Reactions
Bowel Issues, Alternative Treatments, and Life-Saving Support

Since her youngest son, Gavin, was born, Cindy Schultz has kept a meticulous record of his life. Beyond the typical keepsake book of first words and first steps, the Wisconsin mom's records track her son's every doctor's visit, the foods he has eaten, his problematic bowel movements, etc. She can pinpoint precisely when Gavin went from scooting around the floor on his back end, earning him the nickname "Scooter McGavin," to crawling at the late age of fourteen months. And she knows exactly when—at twenty months old—Gavin went from a thriving, communicative child to a withdrawn, self-absorbed boy struck with severe autism. A new mom might keep such detailed written accounts out of the desire to capture every precious moment before it slips away into the next stage of development. But Gavin was Cindy's fifth child. For her, the records have helped her bring order to an otherwise calamitous experience of bouncing between doctors and specialists and searching for answers.

Gavin's book has swelled to 157 typed, single-spaced pages and counting. Some day, when she can no longer care for her son, Cindy hopes to pass along this record of his life, to provide his new caregivers with some insight into how Gavin works—the personal strategies she's learned to help him navigate the world.

It's particularly challenging for parents to understand autism that strikes between a child's first and second years of life, what's known as regressive or late-onset autism, a form of autism that sneaks in and snuffs out a normally developing child's inquisitiveness, playfulness, and previously normally progressing ability to speak and interact. Some 25 percent of autism cases in the US are regressive.[1] It is possible that regressive autism reflects an autoimmune condition in which the body attacks its own cells;[2] this could explain the preponderance of bowel problems in children with autism, a gut-brain axis that has yet to be unraveled.

Cindy's experience raising a son with autism has shaken her confidence in standard medical protocol and the way medical advice is doled out. Cindy had a high fever when Gavin was born after labor was induced at thirty-six weeks. Her blood pressure shot up to 180 over 112, so doctors immediately put her newborn son, who was diagnosed with high bilirubin (a jaundice condition common in newborns) and low blood sugar levels, on antibiotics as a precautionary measure. His weight fell, and they kept him an extra day at the hospital. Then Gavin's test for phenylketonuria (PKU) came back abnormal. All infants are screened at birth for PKU, a genetic disorder that increases the level of phenylalanine, a substance found in all proteins and in some artificial sweeteners, in the blood. If caught early, the proper diet can prevent PKU from leading to developmental problems; if not, the build-up of phenylalanine in a child's body can lead to brain damage, including autism.[3] Gavin's follow-up test came back normal, so PKU was ruled out, but looking back, Cindy wonders if that first test was an indicator of problems to come.

Cindy struggled to receive a proper diagnosis throughout Gavin's early years. While her son was able to say a string of words by eleven months—"Mommy," "Daddy," "Up," "Bye-Bye," and "No-No"—he never seemed to have a normal bowel movement, instead veering between the extremes of constipation and diarrhea. He also never slept through the night and still, at age twelve, very rarely does. But the serious concerns began when Gavin was twenty months old, and the formerly happy, affectionate child morphed from a normally developing boy into one who seemed at odds with the world around him. By the time Gavin turned two, he reacted violently to taking baths. He was constantly moody, throwing tantrums, pacing back and forth through the house, flapping his hands, and dancing on his toes. One day he banged his head repeatedly with his hand and against the floor. Cindy knelt, crying, trying to comfort him, knowing something was terribly wrong inside her son. In the section of Gavin's book titled "Two Years to Three Years," Cindy wrote, "The closer Gavin got to the age of two, it was clear he was not doing normal things":

> May 4, 2000. Gavin saw Dr. Mataczynski at All Saints Health Care. He just said he is in his terrible two's. Gavin was so hyper during that appointment I could not control him. He was like a caged animal in the exam room.
>
> Gavin has never had a problem when we went to Grandma's before but he did not want to go into the kitchen. Later I thought about it and realized how she has very high ceilings and when you talk in that room it echoes and you can hear the clock tick and the refrigerator running. It may have been too much for him to get used to.

At home, the strange behaviors continued. Her son had no interest in children's books, but he would stare, fascinated, at the picture-less pages of a Bible on the family's cocktail table. When Gavin went outside to play, he ignored his toys and stared at the tires of the car parked in the driveway, or rode his tricycle around the court, stopping to study every mailbox along the way. He showed little interest in movies, but was entranced by the credits at a movie's end.

One summer shortly into Gavin's second year, Cindy, her husband Randy, and their older children—Justin, Stephanie, and Tiffany—attended an outdoor festival while the youngest two kids, Meghan and Gavin, stayed with their godparents. Gavin spent nearly the entire time pacing back and forth at the fence in the yard until his parents returned. His behavior drew the attention of a nurse living next door, who later told Cindy and her husband that she suspected Gavin had autism. When Cindy read the description of autism from the nurse's medical journal, there was no doubt in her mind. She took her troubled son to Children's Hospital of Wisconsin in nearby Milwaukee, where they failed to diagnose Gavin for several months, despite the obvious signs. "To this day," Cindy says, "I still have parents coming to my autism support group saying 'Children's Hospital didn't diagnose my child. It took that many more months to get services for my child.' Nowadays, how can they not know what it is? What's their fear? They have to be helped. To be able to get the extra services, they need that label."[4]

Gavin's autism has brought clarity to Cindy's family; in fact, it helped her to recognize the high-functioning characteristics of ASD in both her husband and her eldest son. With Justin in particular, the hallmarks of Asperger's syndrome were unmistakable, once she recognized them. Just as Gavin had an early fascination with books full of words, Justin was once mesmerized by phone books. His mom would give him an old phone book and he would spend hours flipping through the pages and tearing them into long strips. Justin loved *Star Wars* characters and Matchbox cars, too, and he lined them up in a very particular order and requested a new model each week, not wanting to be one piece short of a perfect collection. As Justin grew older, he didn't socialize the way other kids his age did; he had trouble maintaining eye contact and developed just one solid friendship into adulthood. But these traits, while quirky, didn't stand in the way of success for Cindy's oldest son. Instead, when looking for jobs, he found work that required minimal social interaction—loading trucks for United Postal Service and cleaning a local movie theater. By age thirty, Justin had bought his own home, paid his bills promptly each month, and was completely self-reliant. "We never had to help him out with anything," Cindy says.

It was her daughters who first pointed out that their dad had characteristics of Asperger's, too. He pursued his geekier tendencies with obsessive interest, the evidence of which has overtaken the family's basement. There are the ham radios, lined up on basement shelves, and outside, the antennas and towers to support them. Then there are the six computers, in various stages of disrepair, which Randy is in the midst of rebuilding. When he took up an interest in photography one year, he did so fully—building a dark room in yet another basement corner. Even Randy has become convinced, the more he reads about Asperger's, that he fits the description.

The Schultzes live just two miles from the Oak Creek coal-fired power plant, operated by Wisconsin Electric, or We Energies. The plant's sky-high lead and mercury emissions have resulted in the Milwaukee region being ranked in the top 20 percent of dirtiest counties in the US by Scorecard, an online pollution information site managed by the nonprofit Environmental Defense Fund, which compiles data from over 400 scientific and government databases.[5] The power plant expanded to the tune of $2.3 billion amid controversy in early 2010, and the formidable structure with its belching smokestacks now sprawls across 1,000 acres.[6] Forty-five of these acres are covered by a fly ash landfill that holds the dirty, powdered remains of the plant's coal-burning operations. In April 1982, January 1987, and February 2009, the plant was found to be out of compliance with state or federal regulations.[7] According to EPA data, as of 2009 the plant's smokestacks were releasing 23 pounds of lead per year into surrounding air, and nearly 190 pounds of mercury. The plant was also responsible for the release of 36 pounds of lead and 14.6 pounds of mercury into the ground.

Scorecard has a system to help determine the collective impact of these various emissions on human health. Reported releases of chemicals that cause noncancerous health effects are weighted according to their toxicity and exposure potential and converted into pounds of toluene-equivalents (carcinogens are measured separately and converted into pounds of benzene-equivalents). A toluene-equivalent unit serves as a common denominator for comparing noncancer-causing chemical releases; the units indicate the number of pounds of toluene that would have to be released into the air to pose the same approximate level of health risk as the reported release of any certain chemical.[8] Toluene was chosen as the common denominator because it falls in the middle range of noncancer-causing chemicals in terms of toxicity to human health. Using this measurement, Scorecard has ranked the Oak Creek plant, which is responsible for 990,000,000 pounds of toluene-equivalents, first among Milwaukee's most dangerous facilities. The next most dangerous facility, Milwaukee's C&D Technologies Inc., which produces industrial batteries and systems for storing electrical power, releases 750,000,000 pounds of toluene-equivalents.[9]

As recently as June 2006, well water surrounding the Oak Creek Power Plant was found to be polluted with higher-than-allowable levels of a dissolved metal called molybdenum, which has been linked in high exposure levels with liver problems, gout, joint pain, and, in animals, fetal deformities.[10] State regulations allow for 40 micrograms of the metal per liter, but water samples taken from residents' wells near the power plant were found to contain triple that amount in some cases. The Wisconsin Department of Natural Resources told residents not to drink or cook with their water, and We Energies provided bottled water by the caseload to these residents for more than a year while they worked to resolve the problem. The power plant's coal ash landfill was the suspected source of the leaked metals, but answers were in short supply. One affected resident, eighty-four-year-old retiree George Bink, was quoted in the local paper saying, "It's a hush-hush thing: nobody knows anything about [the water contamination] except the people here who're suffering. The electric company has made this a living hell for us out here."[11]

Cindy has been reluctant to point the finger at the power plant in regard to her son's autism. After all, she says, "There are so many kids in our area that don't have autism." She mentions that when they first bought their home in Racine, it was meant to be a starter home. Now, lawn antennas, coal ash, and all, it's clear they don't plan to move. Some friends did move, she said, when the Oak Creek Power Plant expanded and people grew concerned about the black film from the plant's smoky discharge—thick enough to wipe a finger through—that coated the sides of their homes. But Cindy, like many moms who have watched their children change from affectionate and responsive to nearly impossible to reach seemingly overnight, still believes her son's health was damaged by vaccines. His developmental unraveling, she says, tracks with when he received multiple doses of the typical vaccine rounds to prevent diptheria, pertussis, and tetanus (DPT); polio; and haemophilus influenzae type b (Hib), the cause of bacterial meningitis. In recent years, many people have taken issue with the sheer number of vaccines to which children are now subjected. In 1985, kids were vaccinated for just seven diseases; now they are vaccinated for sixteen, for a total of some thirty-seven separate vaccination encounters. Parental discomfort with vaccinations has risen along with the number of administered shots—since the procedure involves holding down a squirming, screaming infant while a nurse injects him in a tender thigh, such discomfort is entirely understandable—giving rise to a generation of "conscientious objectors." Such objectors have decided, against established medical advice, to forgo vaccinations altogether, or to space them out in single-dose administrations.[12]

It is common for parents of children with regressive autism to feel the desire to blame some event for triggering the onset of the disease in their once typically functioning child. For Cindy and many other parents, the coinciding of regressive autism with certain childhood vaccinations left them convinced that their child was somehow overwhelmed by vaccines at a vulnerable time, despite any medical evidence. But it's important, says Dr. Darold A. Treffert, a Wisconsin psychiatrist, author of two books on autism, and consultant on savants for the 1988 Dustin Hoffman film *Rain Man*, to remember that autism is not a single disorder, but a group of disorders "with shared symptoms and a final clinical path." And just as autism has several manifestations, it has a multitude of causes. Dr. Treffert holds that while there is a natural tendency to find blame, and even, in the case of many parents, to cast aspersions on the medical community as a whole following a sudden autism regression, doctors and researchers have been vocal about drug insults to children in the past (alerting the public about the dangers of thalidomide and the use of antidepressants in children, for example) and that they seek, first and foremost, to "raise awareness" and "advocate for a prompt remedy."[13]

As Arizona State's Dr. James Adams exhibited in the aforementioned studies investigating the teeth and baby hair of children with autism, autistic children's bodies do have greater difficulty getting rid of mercury and other heavy metals.[14] Such mercury exposure can come via their mothers' bloodstreams during pregnancy, or in breast milk.[15] And the amount of mercury found in the hair of children with autism in Adams's study "showed a significant correlation" with the number of mercury-containing dental fillings their mothers had,[16] another often overlooked source for the toxic metal.

As noted earlier, Dr. Adams discovered that infants with autism had experienced more ear infections—and thus, more doses of antibiotics—than the average child. Autistic children's decreased ability to excrete mercury normally may be related to their increased exposure to antibiotics during infancy, which disrupts the way the body's intestines work. And the frequent ear infections themselves could be a sign of something amiss with the child's immune system. Normally, bacteria in the intestines convert rapidly absorbed methylmercury into inorganic mercury, which is then excreted. Yeast and *Escherichia coli* (*E. coli*) work in reverse, changing inorganic mercury to methylmercury and preventing its excretion. With increased antibiotics, yeast and *E. coli* are also increased, causing the body to retain more mercury.[17]

Up to 70 percent of children with autism have bowel problems, according to some reports, leading not only to constipation and diarrhea, but to painful bloating and cramping.[18] Outward physical signs include distended bellies, pale complexions, and dark circles under the eyes. But current studies discount the autism-gut problem connection; one 2009 study found no significant differences in stool patterns, color, or consistency, or differences in tendency to have diarrhea or constipation, between children with autism and typical children.[19] The *British Medical Journal* has disavowed any such connection as well; the association, dubbed "autistic enterocolitis" (enterocolitis is a term for an inflamed colon or small intestine) by Andrew Wakefield, has been discredited along with his research.[20]

In any case, there is plenty of evidence that kids with autism have difficulty getting rid of toxic metals. That difficulty could be caused in part by early exposure to antibiotics, but it could also be tied to lower levels of glutathione (GSH), an important antioxidant molecule that helps to control oxidative stress and prevent cell damage by aiding the body in processing medications and cancer-causing compounds, and building DNA and proteins. Oxidative stress happens when the body has an increase in cell-damaging free radicals that can come from any number of sources (including pollution, stress, cigarette smoking, alcohol consumption, cold, and trauma[21]), and GSH acts as the body's natural buffer. Researcher Jill James, the director of the Metabolic Genomics Laboratory at the Arkansas Children's Hospital Research Institute, was the first to discover this breakthrough association between low glutathione levels and autism, finding in one 2004 study that "relative to the control children, the children with autism had . . . significantly higher concentrations" of "oxidized glutathione" or GSSG, which is consistent with "impaired capacity for methylation . . . and increased oxidative stress." Healthy cells and tissues have high levels of GSH, and low levels of GSSG; autistic kids had an almost twofold increase in levels of GSSG, and the ratio of GSH to GSSG "was reduced by 70 percent." Such an abnormal metabolic profile, the study reports, could be due to "a genetic predisposition to environmental agents or conditions that promote oxidative stress . . . in the autistic children."[22] In an e-mail interview, James relates that there are a host of chemicals in the environment that deplete glutathione including "metals (lead, mercury, arsenic, cadmium, aluminum, cobalt), solvents (alcohol, benzene, chlorinated solvents), and industrial chemicals (pesticides, herbicides, PCBs)."

> Although these chemicals are structurally diverse with very different chemical structures, they all have a common mechanism of toxicity which includes glutathione depletion. Because many of these chemicals are ubiquitous in the environment, it is highly likely that we are chronically exposed to multiple chemicals even though they may be below the documented 'safe upper limit.' The problem is that the safe upper limit is defined for each chemical in isolation and it is plausible that there could be an additive effect from multiple simultaneous exposures that could interactively decrease GSH/GSSG detoxification capacity and reach a toxic threshold."[23]

Discovering where these deficiencies lie has helped researchers move beyond looking for the causes of autism to finding ways to minimize its impact. James is involved in research that looks at the role of nutritional supplements that support GSH production and whether such supplements can improve outcomes for kids with autism. Many parents, including the Schultzes, have made steady gains with their children by eliminating certain dietary triggers that seem to aggravate autistic symptoms, including wheat and dairy. Cindy has had Gavin on a gluten-free, casein-free (GFCF) diet for years, and her son is slowly regaining the capacity for language and interaction that he'd lost, benefits she attributes both to a controlled diet and regular behavioral therapy. At age twelve, she counted it as a small victory that Gavin said "Eat up" at a recent meal, words he hadn't said since he was thirteen months old.

Another Midwest mom, Shauna Layton of Indiana, who founded the support group Together in Autism (TIA), relates that her son Hayden Michael had a similar turnaround in language ability when she switched him to a GFCF diet. By age two and a half, Hayden Michael was struggling with ailments including chronic ear infections and bowel problems. He didn't respond to his name, lined up his toys obsessively, demanded strict repetition of daily tasks, and melted down when life intervened. By the time her son was six, Layton had read reams of information about autism treatments and taken charge of his recovery. She began by eliminating dairy. "It was like he was going through detox, he was so addicted to it," she says. After a week without milk, cheese, or other dairy products, he went from saying only a few words to asking "who, what, where, when, and why" questions, she says, and answering them. After six months on a full GFCF diet, Hayden Michael began speaking in full sentences. So Layton removed more potential triggers from his diet—eliminating sugar and yeast, and adding fish oil. "I was so blown away," Layton recalls. "My son was doing all things now to an extreme in a neurotypical manner. I was learning who my son was as he was expressing his likes and dislikes." She cautions that there is no magic cure, "no standard treatment [and] no guarantee for every child." At the same time, she's witnessed plenty of evidence from the many families who belong to her support group that a GFCF diet can unlock the ability to speak in some children with autism—allowing them to finally express how they're feeling. "I get goosebumps every time," Layton says. "Some children have never talked, and now they are saying 'Mom,' 'Dad,' or 'I love you' for the first time."[24]

To date, the positive impacts of eliminating wheat and dairy on autistic behaviors remains largely anecdotal, but the GFCF lifestyle has many vocal advocates, particularly in the alternative health community. Proponents of controlled diets for kids with autism say many of the behaviors kids with autism exhibit, from flapping their hands, to making high-pitched noises, to angry outbursts, may be in part related to their constant discomfort—discomfort they are helpless to articulate. Dr. Kenneth Bock, who treats children with autism with a variety of alternative methods at the Rhinebeck Health Center in New York, says that some of the kids with autism he sees in his practice "look like they come from third-world countries, with bloated bellies and thin extremities." They regularly have inflammation in their colons, as well as "an imbalance of intestinal flora," and that "abnormal instestinal flora overgrowth of anaerobic bacteria or yeast can create abnormal behaviors."[25]

Dr. Bock specializes in chelation therapy, a controversial alternative treatment for both autism and heart disease that the FDA has approved only to treat victims of lead or other heavy metal poisoning. Sometimes chelation involves administering injections of ethylenediaminetetraacetic acid (EDTA) into the blood; the EDTA binds to the heavy metals and allows them to be excreted in the urine. Another chelator, dimercaptosuccinic acid (DMSA), is taken orally, and is available in supplement form online. Adams used DMSA in his study assessing whether the amount of metals excreted by children with autism correlated with the severity of their disorder. After administering DMSA, Adams conducted a regression analysis, which showed that such a correlation did exist. "The regression analysis found that the body burden of toxic metals (as assessed by urinary excretion before and after DMSA) was significantly related to the variations in the severity of autism," the 2009 study notes. "The metals of greatest influence were lead (Pb), antimony (Sb), mercury (Hg), tin (Sn), and aluminum (Al)."[26] Adams's study was the first to establish this connection between metals and the severity of the disorder. "We found children with high levels of toxic metals tended to be much more severely autistic," he says, "and this was incredibly statistically significant. We found that we could explain roughly 45 percent of the severity of autism using the best assessment tool out there, based on the level of toxic metals in these kids. So that was a very, very powerful finding. No one to my knowledge has yet found such a high association of autism with anything."[27] The study also cautioned that it was not just one metal that should raise flags, but various metals acting in concert, concluding, "it is probably best to not overinterpret the results in terms of a particular metal, but to instead interpret them as evidence of the general role of toxic metals in relation to the severity of autism."

Despite its seeming effectiveness and popularity, the process of removing toxic metals using chelation is controversial. Initial worries about chelation concerned the fact the procedure could deplete necessary minerals, like zinc and iron, along with heavy metals, a side effect that could be countered with daily multivitamins. But since so many children with autism have undergone chelation—some estimates indicate the number to be as high as one in twelve—NIMH initiated a study in 2006 to determine chelation's effectiveness as an autism treatment.[28] The trial was abandoned in 2008 after a study published in *Environmental Health Perspectives* revealed that DMSA administered to rats could cause cognitive defects in animals that did not have high levels of metals in their bodies. Those rats that did begin the study with high lead levels, however, showed marked improvements in cognitive functioning after chelation. The study, by Cornell Professor Barbara Strupp, was the first to show that "chelation therapy can reduce behavioral and learning problems due to lead exposure as well as . . . that this type of treatment can have lasting adverse effects when administered in the absence of elevated levels of heavy metals," according to a related release.[29] In light of these risks, the NIMH shut down its chelation study and redirected the funds, stating, "The board determined that there was no clear evidence for direct benefit to the children who would participate in the chelation trial and that the study presents more than a minimal risk."[30] Chelation's troubling past also includes the death of a five-year-old boy with autism in Pennsylvania—a boy who went into cardiac arrest after his doctor administered the wrong EDTA chelator. The boy was given disodium EDTA instead of calcium disodium EDTA—both are clear, colorless, and odorless—but the drug given to the boy fatally robbed his body of calcium, causing his heart to stop beating.[31] It was not the therapy itself, but the medical mix-up that led to his death.

Adams notes that the lack of long-term studies on chelation and the ease of purchasing relatively cheap chelators like DMSA over-the-counter are both problematic. According to Adams, when purchased online, DMSA costs "maybe $100 a month or less, less than almost any treatment out there . . . compared to ABA [applied behavior analysis] therapy [which can cost more than $70,000 per year[32]] it's extremely cheap."[33] Like many alternative autism treatments, chelation continues to hold allure for parents who are increasingly aware of the connection between toxic build-ups and the disorder. But such treatments should only be followed under a physician's direction—a recommendation underscored by the risks identified in Strupp's study. Adams suspects there may be a benefit, someday, to measuring a pregnant woman's heavy metal levels and boosting her detoxification system, particularly for those with low glutathione levels, with supplements like vitamin B-12 and folinic acid (both of which boost glutathione levels and are used in autism treatments). Such detoxing of the mother prior to a baby's birth might, he posits, work to counteract autism arising in the first place, and with it the need for detoxing children.[34]

There are two distinct directions that parents of an autistic child tend to follow as they delve into online research and testimonies: the path of traditional specialists and doctors, or the path of alternative treatments. Those in the first group rely on nearby available services and the ABA mentioned by Adams, in which certain behaviors are reinforced by rewards to improve communication skills, social skills, and basic self-care. The earlier and more intensively a child with autism begins ABA, the better; there are some who respond so well that they are able to effectively participate in a regular classroom after years of the therapy.[35] ABA is used by special education teachers and is widely approved for treating autism.

Sharon Sandifer Holmes, who is trained in reinforcement-based teaching for special needs kids, has adapted it to home life, too. She uses rewards such as computer time to encourage her son James to drink water, take a shower, or complete other tasks he's reluctant to do. Bobbie Gallagher does the same with Austin, who stubbornly resists basic day-to-day tasks. She agrees to let Austin have one of his favorite foods if he agrees to take a bath. For both moms, their children's care is a team effort—a team that involves school specialists, therapists, medical doctors, and, when necessary, intensive neurobehavioral care (as when Austin turns aggressive). Such around-the-clock care is expensive, costing anywhere from $67,000 to $72,000 per year, according to the Harvard School of Public Health.[36] Parents raising a child with autism will spend $4,110 to $6,200 more per year on medical costs than they would for a typical child.[37] Over the course of their lifetime, each person with autism costs society $3.2 million, according to an April 2007 study in *Archives of Pediatrics and Adolescent Medicine*, primarily due to lost productivity and the cost of adult care. Meanwhile, the combined cost for managing autism in both direct and indirect care is estimated to cost society about $35 billion each year.[38] It can be a struggle for parents to obtain insurance coverage for necessary therapies, and those figures don't take into account the impact of sudden emergencies that require parents to leave their jobs to care for their child. For many parents, treating their child's autism has become their full-time job, with any free time they have devoted to autism advocacy through local support groups they join or form themselves.

Alternative treatments can be expensive, too. Cindy, determined to get her son well, has sought out alternative treatments from Defeat Autism Now! (DAN!) approved doctors, physicians who support detoxifying kids with chelation, employing elimination diets like GFCF, and administering dietary supplements, including cod liver oil, melatonin, folic acid, and methyl B-12 injections.[39] These doctors also support biomedical treatments like hyperbaric oxygen therapy, in which patients sit in a pressurized room or submarine-shaped pod and breathe in highly pressurized air that allows them to take in up to three times more oxygen than normal. The increased oxygen circulates through the blood, and, according to the Mayo Clinic, stimulates the body to release "substances called growth factors and stem cells, which promote healing."[40] These chambers are available for home use at costs ranging from $1,500 a month to rent, or up to $20,000 to purchase a large model. They have led to improvements in language and understanding in some children with autism, but it can take forty treatments or more to see such results. One Maine mother, Marty Ann Kelley, bought a hyperbaric oxygen chamber to treat her autistic son, Kenneth, at home, and credits the fact that her eight-year-old is able to talk to the more than 700 hours he has spent inside. Kelley also has her son on a "specific carbohydrate diet," and injects him with methyl B-12 specially ordered from a Florida pharmacy. She has traveled with Kenneth to Costa Rica to the Institute of Cellular Medicine, where he was injected with 24 million stem cells drawn from umbilical cord blood over four days, a treatment she says has brought "lots of results in his cognition and speech." Kelley belongs to Layton's Together in Autism group, which she says has given her the tools and support to take on her son's treatments independently. "We are fanatical about understanding autism, what is causing it, and how to help combat it better every day, week and month," she says. "Being considered 'wacko' by most people, these moms on TIA are the first to understand and are ahead of science and doctors due to their hands-on experience with their autistic children."[41]

While she hasn't gone to such extreme lengths in terms of treatment, Cindy shares Marty Ann Kelley's fanaticism in helping Gavin. She started home schooling him from an early age, and he responds to her better than any specialist she's found. Cindy is determined to make the process easier for other families facing an autism diagnosis, to spare them the early years of frantic research and endless questions. She began the organization Autism Network through Guidance, Education & Life, Inc. (ANGEL, Inc.) in 2000 to help raise money for autism treatments and to provide a family support network, an educational resource, and a social outlet for Wisconsin families struggling to deal with the daily pressure and stress of caring for special needs children. Cindy has seen, firsthand, the toll that autism takes on families. "I have had so many friends going through divorce this year—seven of them," she says. "As hard as you try to keep your marriage intact, it's so difficult when you have special needs in your life. Such a big part of your life gets sucked into it. You're trying to find out as much as you can. And I'm trying to help others in the process."

Even though the disorder seems nearly ubiquitous, dealing with autism can still feel incredibly lonely. Aside from the search for treatments, there are the looks to be endured when one takes a child with autism out in public and the isolation of not knowing other families with an autistic child, all underscored with a pervasive fear: not knowing what to do, and not knowing what you may have done, or are doing, wrong.

When autism was first discovered, mothers were blamed first. "Fifty years ago," says Adams, "everyone believed that autism was due to mothers hating their children."[42] During the 1950s and 1960s, the prevailing medical wisdom regarding autism was the "refrigerator mother" theory, which posited that children were autistic because their mothers were "frigid," withholding necessary love and affection. The theory came from one man: the child psychologist Bruno Bettelheim, who was born in Austria and suffered in a Nazi concentration camp, and who believed that the behavioral characteristics evident in children with autism were akin to those seen in prisoners under their Nazi guards.[43] Dr. Hertz-Picciotto of UC Davis says the "refrigerator mother" theory dealt a devastating blow to autism research. "I think the entire scientific community was derailed by the publications in the 1960s that autism was really the result of bad parenting practices and that put a blame on the parents' attitude," she says. "That dominated the scientific community for several decades and has basically set us back."[44]

Though Bettelheim's theory has been utterly discredited, mothers' sense of blame and their fear that they are doing too much or too little have been difficult to shake. In Bobbie Gallagher's case, after she had poured so much effort into discovering the cause for the elevated number of autism cases in her area, she was left feeling betrayed; she felt that people in her community would rather live with the uncertainty than hurt their property values. After the investigators left, Bobbie wondered if her efforts had even been worthwhile. She says, "The sad part for us is when you're doing this, in addition to dealing with autism, is having people you really trust come and say 'We believe in this information you are giving us and want to help you do something about it,' and to find out later you probably shouldn't have trusted them. That they had no intention of finding the problem."

Support groups—whether online or in their communities—are the only things keeping many mothers of children with autism from cracking under the constant pressure. Sharon says the support group for parents with autistic children at her son's Bridgeport school has "made a world of difference" in helping her feel accepted and understood. Mothers who have joined Together in Autism online often relate that they were led there by feelings of isolation and uncertainty, and had nowhere else to turn. One, Kristi Hogg, who lives in a small, rural Tennessee town, and whose younger daughter, Mayci, has autism, said that she felt "alone for eight long years" before she came across TIA's website. She calls herself a "research junky," who spends long hours reading about various autism treatments online, and says, "Together in Autism's site, their Yahoo group and other Yahoo groups have been a lifesaver for me for helping my daughter."[45]

Layton, TIA's founder, says that parents with autism undergo a strenuous amount of judgment from family members, community members, and even doctors. "Regardless of what therapy or treatment they use," she says, "there is difficulty with it in general. In a lot of cases there are people close to them that do not agree with their choices for their child, feel pity for them, judge them, even believe that if it were their child they would not behave in such a manner—or who do not take part in their child's life due to fear," she says. "That is when a support system such as ours is so vital. . . . We are here to help."

The more mothers learn about autism causes and the wide range of available treatments, the more they feel empowered to take action on behalf of their children and to move beyond the self-defeating blame. Raising a child—or children—with autism is an exhausting undertaking, emotionally, psychologically, and financially. Making it work is not a one-woman or even two-parent operation, and support services, wherever they exist, are leading moms and dads to trust their instincts, to try different treatments, to stand up for their kids, and to share their milestones and failures in a place that doesn't judge them for circumstances they cannot control.

"You're thinking you're the only one out there," Sharon says. "James does some odd stuff sometimes, but there are other people going through the same thing."

FIVE

Birth Complications
Weighing the Risks of Inductions, Medications,
and Early Cord Clamping

Like many mothers of autistic children, Cindy's life now centers around autism. Almost daily, she posts links to news stories related to autism on her Facebook page. Some are horror stories: an autistic child forced to play in a cage; a student with autism bitten by a substitute teacher; a desperate California grandmother who fatally shot her autistic grandson and herself. Other posts involve new medical and dietary treatments for autism: how service dogs have been used to reduce stress in autistic children; the benefits of acupuncture; ways to improve picky eating to encourage healthy diets. And there are plenty of stories that point to concerns with the medical industry and vaccine makers, and encouragements for anyone feeling alone in their struggles with autism to join her group and find the support they've been missing. Offline, Cindy organizes fundraisers—including a controversial "rifle raffle" for autism—and social outings like bowling nights for families with kids on the spectrum. Cindy is the definition of a tireless advocate, and jokes that she could see herself being diagnosed with ADHD, saying, "I'm go-go-go and nothing slows me down."

She keeps up with the latest research, too, and when a new finding seems to fit her own experience, she wonders if maybe this is the one that might unlock her own personal autism mystery. She knows that of her five children, Gavin had the most complicated birth, because her own health was compromised in ways it hadn't been before. She took the medication methyldopa (an antihyperintensive drug that relaxes blood vessels) during the pregnancy to counteract her high blood pressure; her labor was induced with pitocin; and, of course, she was older than she was when she had her other children. A study done in Australia and published in 2004 found a correlation between complications during childbirth, older mothers, and autism. That study revealed that children with autism born in Western Australia between 1980 and 1995 were more likely to have had difficult births—near-miscarriages, epidural use, fetal distress, birth by Caesarean section (C-section), and an Apgar score (the infant test that provides a quick snapshot of initial health) lower than six. The study concluded that "Autism is unlikely to be caused by a single obstetric factor," but rather, "The increased prevalence of obstetric complications among autism cases is most likely due to the underlying genetic factors or an interaction of these factors with the environment."[1]

One of the study's lead researchers, Dr. Emma Glasson from the University of Western Australia's School of Population Health, said that her study was unique in that it involved "a large cohort" and "good quality data," but it left many unanswered questions regarding how birth complications and autism might be connected. "Among my study and others, there has not yet been a single pre-, peri-, or postnatal factor that has been positively associated with autism on its own," Glasson says. Despite the large number of participants—465 children diagnosed with autism compared with 481 siblings and 1,313 random controls—she says that, "[the study] still didn't find any predictive factors for autism. Instead it found that as a group, children with autism experienced more difficulties in utero, but this pattern did not fit all the children with autism, and the pattern also was common to some children without a diagnosis. Certainly this is a puzzle," she adds, "and further research is being done on genetics and finer epidemiology (such as dividing the cases by other factors like intellectual disability) to understand the patterns better. This might help us understand why the patterns are present and how the difficulties experienced are related to the diagnosis."[2]

An earlier study conducted by the University of California, San Diego's School of Medicine found an association between autism and birth complications such as uterine bleeding during pregnancy and infant hyperbilirubinemia, or jaundice, a build-up of bilirubin (a brownish-yellow substance found in bile) in the blood, leading to yellow-looking skin in newborns. Mothers of autistic children were also more likely to have induced or prolonged labors, which the study explained may lead to fetal compromise in "the form of asphyxia, infection, or head trauma from prolonged pressure—all of which may have lasting neurologic consequences." There were other similarities found among mothers who gave birth to a child with autism. These mothers had "significantly lower" incidences of "vaginal infection, smoking and contraceptive use" when compared with the general population. Researchers surmised that differences in education levels among the mothers of autistic children may explain these findings. For instance, they wrote: "Incidence of vaginal infection increases with multiple partners, partners with sexually transmitted diseases, and poor hygiene—all of which occur at a higher incidence in lower socioeconomic populations." The study concluded that there appeared to be an association between "unfavorable events in pregnancy, delivery, and the neonatal phase and the pervasive developmental disorders," but that "Additional studies are needed to corroborate and strengthen these associations, as well as to determine the possibility of an underlying unifying pathological process."[3] Multiple studies looking for connections between obstetrics practices or traumatic birth events and autism have reached similar conclusions.

Researchers and doctors are paying closer attention to drugs that have been approved for use during pregnancy and standard obstetrics practices around the birth itself. When determining whether to prescribe a drug, ob-gyns must weigh its benefits to the mother against the risks it may pose to the developing fetus. Such determinations are never easy, and, in the past, have led to tragic medical missteps, such as the widespread birth defects in the 1960s that came about as a result of thalidomide being prescribed to treat morning sickness.

Dr. Michael Merzenich, a pioneer in brain plasticity research, and his fellow researchers at the University of Mississippi studied selective serotonin reuptake inhibitors (SSRIs), antidepressants that have been an accepted treatment for pregnant women and breastfeeding mothers suffering from depression for the past twenty years. SSRIs work by preventing a receptor in the brain from reabsorbing the neurotransmitter serotonin. Commonly prescribed SSRI medications include Prozac, Celexa, Zoloft, Paxil, and Lexapro. Antidepressants are now the most prescribed class of medications in the US, according to findings in the *Archives of General Psychiatry*; as of 2009, 10.12 percent of the US population was taking antidepressants, a 75 percent jump from 1996.[4] Of course, depression itself is a danger to new mothers and can negatively impact their ability to bond with and care for newborns. "We can't have a depressed mother," Dr. Merzenich says. "But the problem is the antidepressants have impacts on brains. And they have impacts both when they're delivered prenatally in the placental blood, and also when delivered postnatally through nursing." In studies with rats, Dr. Merzenich and his team found that SSRIs administered at doses equivalent to those given to both pregnant and nursing mothers "changed the course of development of the brain of the rat." He adds that SSRIs are just one drug of concern among many that are given to pregnant women or to nursing mothers. "My guess is that there's another whole messy set of contributors . . . to the increasing risk of autism," Merzenich says. "Self-administered [drugs] are affecting fetal development."[5]

His concerns were borne out in July 2011 when the *Archives of General Psychiatry* published the results of a study looking at how SSRIs taken prior to and during pregnancy impacted a mother's likelihood of giving birth to a child with autism. Researchers in California looked at 298 children diagnosed with ASD and their mothers, as well as 1,507 randomly selected control children and their mothers. Mothers who took SSRIs during the year before delivery were twice as likely to give birth to a child with autism, "with the strongest effect associated with treatment during the first trimester." No such association was found between non-SSRI antidepressants and autism. But the authors of the antidepressant study caution that "the fraction of cases of ASD that may be attributed to use of antidepressants by the mother during pregnancy is less than 3% in our population, and it is reasonable to conclude that prenatal SSRI exposure is very unlikely to be a major risk factor for ASD." As Dr. Merzenich noted, researchers here concluded that "The potential risk associated with exposure must be balanced with the risk to the mother or fetus of untreated mental health disorders."[6]

The steady rise in autism cases beginning in the 1980s, a phenomenon that molecular biologist Richard Lathe, author of *Autism, Brain and Environment*, has dubbed "new phase autism," also tracks with the regular obstetrics practice of umbilical cord clamping immediately following birth. Cutting the umbilical cord early—as quickly as fifteen seconds after delivery—became standard medical practice in the 1980s, as it was believed to reduce postpartum hemorrhage,[7] the leading cause of maternal death worldwide. Some 500,000 women in third world countries die each year after giving birth; many of these deaths occur within the first four hours after delivery, and a quarter of these deaths come as a result of hemorrhaging.[8] It has become clear, however, that these outcomes are not tied to delayed cord clamping, but to improper or inadequate medical care during and following delivery. Active management of labor, in which a "prophylactic oxytocic"— pitocin—is delivered after the cord is clamped (often early) to aid in placental delivery, has been shown to reduce blood loss and the risk of post partum hemorrhage.[9] And while early cord clamping reduces the risk of jaundice in infants, a 2008 study that examined 11 trials of 2,989 mothers and their babies found that delaying cord clamping "for at least two to three minutes seems not to increase the risk of postpartum haemorrhage" and "can be advantageous for the infant by improving iron status which may be of clinical value particularly in infants where access to good nutrition is poor . . ."[10]

There's increasing evidence that cord clamping should be delayed— even by just a few minutes—to help prevent possible damage to the infant. When the umbilical cord is clamped immediately, reports Dr. Judith S. Mercer, the director of the University of Rhode Island College of Nursing Nurse-Midwifery Program, it "can reduce the red blood cells an infant receives at birth by more than 50 percent, resulting in potential short-term and long-term neonatal problems."[11] Meanwhile, delayed cord clamping provides definite benefits for newborns, including less likelihood of anemia (via the improved iron status), increased blood flow to organs, and higher body temperatures.[12] In a large clinical trial funded by the National Institute of Nursing Research, Dr. Mercer found that delayed cord clamping had another benefit, specifically for male infants: after controlling for other factors, she found that male infants whose cord clamping was delayed had higher motor scores. In an interview with the research blog Science & Sensibility, Dr. Mercer said, "Our study suggested that delayed cord clamping may be protective against motor delay in preterm male infants."[13]

Blood carries oxygen and carbon dioxide from the mother to her baby and back through the umbilical cord and the placenta, a process that supports the fetus' developing organs. The mother's placenta handles the delivery of oxygen and the removal of carbon dioxide, so during pregnancy the fetus doesn't use its lungs for breathing. At the crucial moment of birth, the circulation changes very quickly: a massive increase in blood is sent to the baby's lungs, opening passageways that allow the baby to breathe. The infant's first cry is a clear indication that the fluids in the baby's lungs have been expelled and the air sacs have been opened to initiate normal breathing. But with immediate cord clamping, that needed reservoir of extra blood for the lungs is cut off. The baby must instead draw blood away from other vital organs, a process that could potentially result in a state of oxygen deprivation. It also deprives the newborn of the critical iron supplies needed to make hemoglobin, the blood-borne protein that delivers oxygen to the lungs. "The baby can't absorb iron in its young life very effectively," says Dr. Merzenich. In response to concerns about iron deficiencies following early cord clamping, parents are now routinely told to supplement breastfeeding with iron-containing infant drops and infant formulas and cereals that typically come fortified with iron.

Dr. Merzenich notes that medical practice is beginning to move toward waiting a few minutes before clamping.

> It's shocking to me that the obstetrics practice moved away from the natural—trying to outsmart Mother Nature, as it were—to adopting a very unnatural strategy of cutting the cord in a few tenths of seconds after delivery. All this monitoring occurs that reassures the obstetrician that things are great, but in fact the effectiveness of the oxygenation of the tissues of the body are going to be impeded. You've just down-regulated all of the metabolic processes for the first six months of the life of the child because of what you've done in those first few tenths of seconds. I'm not saying that this is a cause [of autism], and I'm not saying that I know it is a contributing cause. I'm saying when you see something like this that occurs across this

time period, in which we know that the incidence [of autism] is rising, it should be investigated.[14]

It's known that oxygen deprivation has dangerous consequences on
the brain's proper development and functioning at any age. Hypoxia, an
inadequate oxygen supply to the body's cells, can happen when a baby's
brain is denied oxygen due to a poorly developed circulatory system, or
in adults following a stroke, a serious seizure, excessive smoke inhalation
(as in the case of a fire), drug overdose, or drowning. Hypoxia is the most
common cause of brain damage among small and premature infants;
the resulting low pH levels in the umbilical cord blood—making it too
acidic—have been linked to cerebral palsy,[15] a condition in which brain
injuries lead to tightened muscles and joints, muscle weakness, paralysis,
speech problems, digestive problems, and twisting, jerking movements
of the hands, feet, arms, and legs. And a 2000 study found that hypoxia-
related complications during birth "significantly increased the odds of
early-onset schizophrenia."[16]

If cord clamping plays a role in autism cases, it could also help to
explain the mysterious lack of autism cases in the Amish community.
Former *United Press International* reporter Dan Olmsted, who now
edits the Age of Autism website, and others have attempted to link the
lack of autism among the Amish to the community's general refusal to
vaccinate children.[17] But Dr. Merzenich hypothesizes that it has more to
do with the Amish's traditional birth experiences—including delayed
cord clamping. The same theory, he suggests, might help explain the
unusually high rates of autism among Somali families living in Minnesota.[18] These families did not practice early cord clamping in their
home country, but it has become the rule in this immigrant community. In 2008 the rate of autism among Somali children in Minnesota
was found to be two nearly seven times the rate of autism among other
three- and four-year-olds. While Somali children represented just six
percent of the school population in Minneapolis, they comprised 17

percent of those enrolled in early childhood autism programs in the city's schools in 2008.[19] Panicked parents felt blindsided by a disease they did not well understand, and one that seemed to have targeted their community.[20] Autism has had a similar impact on Somali immigrants in Sweden, occurring in Somali populations at three to four times the rate of autism in other populations. In fact, Somalis living in Sweden refer to autism as "the Swedish disease." Some have theorized that a vitamin D deficiency may play a role, thinking that by moving to regions with less sun than their native African country, and living in apartment buildings as opposed to family compounds, they were getting far less vitamin D than their bodies—and their children's developing brains—needed.[21] Predominantly Muslim, the Somali immigrant women living in new countries were more likely to be nearly fully covered at all times, in addition to struggling with the stress of adjustment and the change in diet. But Dr. Merzenich believes that cord clamping deserves careful consideration as a risk factor, since "clamping follows *placental* [author's emphasis] delivery in Somalia, while the cord has been clamped without delay as a general practice in Minnesota [and in countries practicing westernized medicine, including Sweden]."[22] When researchers compared the outcomes of children born following early and late (two minutes or later) cord-clamping in countries with low infant mortality rates (including the US, Canada, Germany, the UK, and Sweden), moderate infant mortality rates (including Argentina and Libya), and higher infant mortality rates (including Egypt, Guatemala, India, and Mexico), they found that "delaying clamping of the umbilical cord for at least two minutes after birth consistently improved both the short- and long-term hematologic and iron status of full-term infants." Most importantly, they concluded, "the beneficial effects of late cord clamping appear to extend beyond the early neonatal period" with a significant reduction in the risk of anemia and having deficient iron stores at two and three months of age. They recommended, based on their findings, "a minimum delay of two minutes before clamping the umbilical cord following birth for all full-term newborns."[23]

Not all researchers are in agreement about the potential consequences of early cord clamping. Jill James, who discovered the link between low glutathione levels and autism, believes that since the infant is breathing independently at the time the umbilical cord is cut, the theory of oxygen deprivation does not make sense.[24] However, James does not address the research pointing to the role early clamping plays in early iron deficiency in newborns. The human brain needs iron to develop properly; iron helps to form a fatty insulation around nerves, and that insulation allows the brain's electrical signals to move rapidly. Dr. Betsy Lozoff, a behavioral/developmental pediatrician at the University of Michigan, and a leading expert on iron deficiency on infant behavior, has found that the impacts of low iron on the brains of infants persists into adulthood. She has found that in lab animals, iron levels correlate with the amount of dopamine and serotonin in the brain—chemicals that help the brain send and receive signals. In an interview with the National Scientific Council on the Developing Child, Lozoff said her studies showed that children with severe iron deficiency in infancy had lower motor skills that remained lower over time; they had poorer social and emotional development, including more anxiety, depression, and inattention; by ages eleven to fourteen they had twice the rate of repeating a grade as children with proper iron levels as infants; and they had significantly lower test scores than other children, a gap that widened over time. Most worrisome was that even after a year of treatment with iron supplements, the early incidence of iron deficiency was not corrected. "In Chile, we're finding that even after treatment for a year with iron drops, children who suffered iron-deficiency anemia as infants have evidence of brain differences 10 years later," Lozoff said in the interview. "Using electrophysiologic tests, we've been able to 'look' into their brains and find that electrical signals move more slowly through their auditory and visual systems. Both the Costa Rican adolescents at 19 years and the Chilean children at 10 years who were treated for severe, chronic iron deficiency in infancy do worse on higher-level cognitive tests."[25]

Iron, as well as selenium, deficiencies make the body more susceptible to toxic build-up of heavy metals. When people are low in iron, for example, they are more likely to have elevated levels of lead in their blood. Researcher Tappan Audya found that one-third of children with autism were deficient in selenium. In *Autism, Brain and the Environment* Richard Lathe writes that "The element [selenium] is increasingly depleted in the diets of some humans, particularly in Europe." Selenium, he notes in the book, helps prevent mercury toxicity; when selenium levels are low, there's evidence of greater "neurological damage induced by methylmercury." Dietary deficiencies may be responsible for acting together with increased exposure to heavy metals and pollutants to cause higher autism rates.[26]

Another common obstetrics practice that has been called into question is increased use of ultrasounds throughout pregnancies, which became standard medical practice beginning in the 1970s. However, a 2009 study involving children born between 1995 and 1999 enrolled in the Kaiser Permanente healthcare system, controlling for factors like maternal age, education, and child's gender, showed no increased risk for autism in relation to number of ultrasounds performed in general or during any particular trimester.[27] The widespread use of pitocin, on the other hand, could be cause for greater concern. Pitocin, a synthetic hormone that mimics the natural hormone oxytocin, is used to induce labor and to speed it up by increasing contractions, but its potential health impacts on infants are not fully understood. Oxytocin has an important relationship with human social interaction. It is released when mothers breastfeed, and also during orgasms, and produces a euphoric state that promotes bonding. It stimulates milk production in lactating mothers, assists in uterine contractions necessary for birth, and, through its release during breastfeeding, promotes the special attachment mothers feel toward their infants, encouraging necessary caregiving.[28] It was once thought that oxytocin's only role was in maternal bonding and lactation, but further study has found oxytocin to be important in helping people trust one another, combat stress, and seek out social support when feeling scared or isolated.[29] In males, oxytocin is present during ejaculation and aids in sperm transport.

When the synthetic hormone pitocin is administered to induce or speed up labor, it produces sharp, fast, painful contractions, accelerating the delivery process and doubling the likelihood that the experience will end in a C-section. Induced labors, along with C-sections, which now account for one third of all births, are on the rise in the US, occurring in 34 percent of single live deliveries in 2009,[30] up from 10 percent of deliveries in 1990.[31] Induction of labor can be a good and necessary procedure when natural childbirth is delayed long past the due date, but in many cases, it actually causes women to give birth early, before their due dates, as happened with Cindy. And pitocin use to speed up labors—shortening deliveries by about two and a half hours on average—as opposed to merely inducing labors, has become nearly ubiquitous in many hospital delivery rooms, particularly for those hospitals that practice a procedure known as "active management of labor." In an editorial accompanying a 2010 study published in *Obstetrics & Gynecology*, Dr. Caroline Signore of the Eunice Kennedy Shriver National Institute for Child Health and Human Development writes, "We must remember that incautious use and timing of interventions—particularly in elective cases—can lead to unnecessarily poorer outcomes for women and newborns."[32]

In adults, pitocin has a short half-life and does not cross the blood-brain barrier, but its impact on newborns is not as clearly understood. An exhaustive study from 2003 connecting the majority of existing research on oxytocin use and its consequences by C. Sue Carter of the University of Illinois at Chicago finds that, "[h]ospitals that adhere to a procedure known as 'active management of labor' may recommend exogenous OT [synthetic oxytocin, or pitocin] for virtually every woman in labor. The use of OT has become so widespread that there is a tendency to assume that its effects are well known and benign, and increased use and even higher doses have been recommended, in some cases in an attempt to reduce the need for Caesarean section." But as Carter reveals, research conducted on animals, particularly prairie voles, shows marked changes in development as a result of early oxytocin exposure. "During development," she writes, "exposure to peptides and steroids [oxytocin is a synthetic hormone that acts as a peptide, or set of amino acids, in the body] may reprogram the nervous system, altering thresholds for sociality, emotionality and aggression." Neonatal stress, she adds, (which may come as the result of a difficult, induced, or surgical birth) can also contribute to an altered OT system. The report notes, "During birth, the levels of circulating oxytocin and vasopressin rise." Vasopressin is another hormone that influences social development and may be given intravenously during childbirth for extremely low birth weight, at-risk babies. "So either an elective Caesarean (which prevents occurrence of these enhancements) or a complicated delivery (which elongates the period during which these high levels occur) may expose the brain and body of the child to a completely different vasopressin/OT signal." This disruption may vary significantly from one childbirth to another depending on specific birth events.[33]

What is known is that there is clearly something amiss with the way the bodies of children with autism produce or process oxytocin. Dr. Eric Hollander, a leading psychiatrist and principal investigator with the National Institutes of Health's Studies for the Advancement of Autism Research and Treatment program, said, "studies in children have found [oxytocin] abnormalities in the plasma levels, and the subgroup of children with autism who are the most socially aloof tend to have the lowest levels of oxytocin."[34]

The fact that oxytocin works differently in males may help to explain the higher incidence of autism seen in males. A 2001 study that found a relationship between lower levels of oxytocin in children with autism looked only at boys, recruited from autism schools and support groups from Massachusetts and Connecticut, "because of the low incidence of autism in girls and the resultant difficulty in obtaining a gender-balanced sample." (Autism is on the rise among girls, but boys still make up the large majority of cases. However, there's increasing speculation that girls with autism—who are less likely to exhibit aggressive behaviors and more likely to be written off as merely "odd"—are being diagnosed later than boys, or not diagnosed at all.[35]) A 2001 study found that oxytocin levels were lower in the blood samples of the twenty-eight boys with autism they looked at, and levels of the precursors to oxytocin—peptides collectively referred to as OT-X—were higher, suggesting that these kids' bodies could not properly process the peptides to their active, useful form. This activity would normally occur in the neurons, suggesting, researchers write, "that there are changes in brain oxytocin processing in autistic children." They theorized that those changes were "probably the result of genetic defects,"[36] though it has since become clear that other insults or events during childbirth could also disrupt this system.

The increased use of pitocin is one likely suspect. When it comes to the role of pitocin in altering the body's oxytocin levels, Dr. Hollander writes, "There has been speculation that induction of labor with pitocin somehow disrupts the oxytocin systems of genetically susceptible neonates, ultimately leading to the social deficits of autism." He adds, "A firm association of autism with this use of pitocin has not been established. While a high incidence of pitocin-induced labor has been observed in a clinical population of autistic patients, another survey found no such relationship."[37] Dr. Hollander observes that more studies related to pitocin and autism are needed, and that such a relationship may, in the end, be difficult to prove definitively. It's a chicken-and-egg situation. Do the difficulties already present in the child with autism necessitate the use of pitocin-induced labor? Or is the pitocin-induced labor itself playing a role in the later development of autism? The answer is important, since induced labors happen for a number of reasons that have nothing to do with medical necessity; rather, healthcare providers or pregnant women may choose earlier births for "comfort or convenience" under the belief that delivering a few weeks early will have little impact on the health of themselves or their child.

One theory suggests that by administering pitocin during labor, a child's own system of oxytocin production is disrupted—that the chemical intruder somehow diminishes the infant's natural hormone production or hormone-binding ability, leaving them deficient. Because pitocin can cross the placenta and could impact an "underdeveloped or stressed infantile blood brain barrier at birth," says Roy U. Rojas Wahl with the Initiative for Molecular Studies in Autism in *Medical Hypotheses*, "[A] causal connection between OT excess and behavioral disorders such as autism can be supported from a molecular perspective."[38] And early research with animal models suggests that while oxytocin deficiencies may not provide the full answer to what's causing autism, something amiss with the body's process of secreting the hormone into the blood where it binds to receptors "may account for several features of autism," specifically behaviors such as social withdrawal, lack of trust, poor communication, and repetitive behaviors.

A 2011 study from Colorado State University, meanwhile, found a compelling association between pitocin use during childbirth and the subsequent development of ADHD. The researcher examined the hospital records of 172 people ages three to twenty-five from different regions of the country and looked at twenty-one potential predictors of them later developing ADHD, including obstetric complications, family history of ADHD, and gender. Pitocin exposure jumped out. "Results revealed a strong predictive relationship between perinatal pitocin exposure and subsequent childhood ADHD onset," the study concluded. ADHD occurred in 67.1 percent of those exposed to pitocin during childbirth, as opposed to 35.6 percent for those who were not exposed. While the length of the pitocin exposure, overall gestation, and labor length had some correlation with later ADHD as well, the correlation was strongest with exposure to pitocin itself.[39] There is significant overlap between ADHD and autism, including social and language difficulties and repetitive behaviors, and certain characteristics of ADHD, such as impulsivity and hyperactivity, are often seen in children on the spectrum. One report found that "symptoms consistent with ADHD are present in a significant proportion of children with a PDD [pervasive developmental disorder, indicating autism] . . . anything between 50+ and 75%."[40] Treatments for the two disorders are quite different—kids with ADHD respond better to medications and show greater improvements in abilities over time—but autism and ADHD share many symptoms and may both, in fact, be present in the same child.[41]

The latest research shows that problems with oxytocin production or its reception in children with autism may be epigenetic, the result of a chemical intrusion or other environmental factor silencing a critical gene early in the process of fetal development. A 2010 study published in *BMC Medicine* suggests that sometime very early in gestation molecules called methyl groups bind to the DNA of an individual with autism, preventing the expression of the gene tied to oxytocin reception.[42] "Excess methylation of the oxytocin receptor could render people with autism less sensitive to the social hormone's effects," reflected Dr. Christopher Fisher in *The Behavioral Medicine Report*.[43]

Oxytocin is showing promise as a potential treatment for autism, lending even more weight to the importance of this hormone in understanding the disorder. In one study, researchers found that after giving kids with autism an inhaled form of oxytocin, they exhibited significant improvements in social behaviors. The kids were observed playing a game with a ball; those who had been given oxytocin were more likely to return the ball to the most cooperative player—in other words, they were able to distinguish friendlier playmates. These same kids also showed more attentiveness to photos of faces, and looked more often at the eyes; kids with autism given a placebo were more likely to look at mouths or to look away.[44] Eye contact is critical in social interaction and is a major difficulty for kids with autism. Cindy has said that even her oldest son, Justin, who has Asperger's, has struggled with maintaining eye contact, and it has hampered his ability to form friendships. "It's not like we have to stare in somebody's eyes the whole time we talk to them," Cindy says, "but in the same breath, you want to acknowledge the fact that 'I'm going to be talking to you.' I may glance away, but I look back at you to acknowledge that 'Yes, we are communicating.' [Kids with autism] just don't do that. It's hard for them to look at the person while they're talking."[45] Without that interaction—and that affirmation—it's difficult for parents, too, to develop the same closeness and bond with their autistic children. On a very basic, primal level, particularly in those early years, parents, need to feel that what they say and do matters.

Oxytocin treatment for autism is in the early stages, and because there are no long-term studies, there is some concern about how effective it is in treating autism's symptoms over a lifetime. Its effects are short-lived; although an oxytocin spray or injection may help a person with autism respond to immediate behavioral treatments or tasks, those benefits won't last.[46] Other natural autism therapies that induce the body to produce oxytocin can bring similar benefits without the related worries of side effects or potential long-term harm. These include activities that function like massage, such as lying under a mattress, rolling in a gym mat, or using Dr. Temple Grandin's innovative "squeeze machine," a device that squeezes a person between two thick pads, providing the calming effects of deep-touch pressure without the anxiety associated with a human-administered massage.

Dr. Grandin—an animal scientist, professor, author, and world-famous autism self-advocate whose life was captured with incredible sincerity by actress Claire Danes in *Temple Grandin*, an Emmy-winning HBO movie—has been able to tell the world at large, perhaps better than anyone, what it is to think and feel as a person with autism. Grandin's perception of the world through vivid, visual depictions has also allowed her to understand animals—through both a lifetime of study and an intuitive sense—the way most humans can't. In *Animals in Translation: Using the Mysteries of Autism to Decode Animal Behavior*, a book she co-wrote with Dr. Catherine Johnson, Grandin writes of yet another way humans increase the positive benefits of the social hormone oxytocin—petting a dog. "A dog's oxytocin levels rise when his owner pets him, and petting a dog raises the owner's oxytocin too," the authors write. "I'm sure that's one reason why so many people have dogs in the first place. I don't think anyone has researched this yet, but I suspect we'll find that dogs make humans into nicer people and better parents."[47] A 2009 study from the University of Japan confirmed that interaction with a pet dog in play sessions that involved prolonged eye contact resulted in a 20 percent jump in participants' oxytocin levels.[48] This boost of oxytocin has been found to enhance mood and feelings of trust and well-being and to alleviate anxiety. A study from the College of Veterinary Medicine at Washington State University found that children with autism "exhibited a more playful mood, were more focused, and were more aware of their social environments when in the presence of a therapy dog."[49] Another study published in the *American Journal of Occupational Therapy* found that when such therapy incorporated animals among children aged seven to thirteen with autism, "the children demonstrated significantly greater use of language and significantly greater social interaction . . . when compared to sessions using exclusively standard occupational therapy techniques."[50]

Finding ways to bring children with autism out of their shells—to develop the social interactions like eye contact, willingness to respond to others, and awareness of emotional cues that most of us take for granted—is a challenge. Environmental triggers can work to undo the body's natural brain and hormone development, from zygote to fetus to infant to toddler, but introduced oxytocin-boosting supplements and therapies can also work to alleviate the symptoms that make living with ASD so challenging. Of course the goal is to prevent autism from arising in the first place, and to minimize the exposures that might be acting as triggers.

The 2010 report "Deadly Delivery: The Maternal Healthcare Crisis in the USA" by Amnesty International reveals that the US has an abysmal record when it comes to ensuring the health and wellbeing of women in delivery rooms, particularly if those women happen to be black or minority. Despite spending more than any other country on health care, the number of women who die as a result of childbirth complications in the US has climbed from 6.6 deaths for every 100,000 live births in 1987 to 13.3 deaths for every 100,000 live births in 2006.[51] Those figures put the US behind forty other countries when it comes to maternal mortality rates. And African American women are four times as likely as white women to die as a result of childbirth, as they come to hospitals with a range of disadvantages such as lack of prenatal care, lack of insurance, and lack of proper medical care following births. The rise of C-sections is a major factor in these shocking death rates. "Many women are not given a say in decisions about their care and do not get enough information about the signs of complications and the risks of interventions, such as inducing labor or C-sections," the report finds. "The risk of death following C-sections is more than three times higher than for vaginal births."[52]

As is the case with the untested health-disrupting chemicals circulating freely in our homes and products, medical interventions surrounding childbirth, including the widespread use of pitocin to induce and accelerate labor, have become so commonplace that there's a built-in assumption that such procedures have been tested for safety. But as C. Sue Carter writes, nothing could be further from the truth. "[D]uring childbirth women and potentially their infants may be exposed to varying amounts of exogenous [external] and endogenous [internal] hormone, analgesics, anesthesia, the stressful side effects of the birth experience, and in some cases surgery. Although such complex manipulations are routine in modern obstetrics, little is known regarding the possible consequences of such treatments."[53] Autism is one of many health and developmental disorders on the rise thanks in part to our collective hubris in, as Dr. Merzenich calls it, "outsmarting Mother Nature."

SIX

Our Chemical World
The Long Reach of Plastics and Pesticides

It is hard to imagine life without plastic. It is everywhere simultaneously, seen and unseen. Plastic is present in schoolyard floors and playground furniture; baby toys, bottles, strollers, and sippy cups; snack containers and microwaveable dishes; the lining of soup cans and cans of infant formula; and the packaging of nearly everything. Plastic is cheap, it's durable, and it preserves food well. Kids have to try fairly hard to hurt their siblings with a plastic mallet, as opposed to, say, a wooden one. But the chemicals that are used to make these plastic products come loose over time and are released into the air, the water, and the soil. They are inadvertently eaten. These chemicals wind up in our bloodstream and our milk supply; they are passed from mother to child. Plastic, accumulated in massive quantities year after year, leaves a toxic legacy.

The oceans have become a giant dumping ground for our plastic remains. Nowhere is this more evident than the "Great Pacific Garbage

Patch": 100 million tons of trash trapped by circulating underwater currents between California, Hawaii, and Japan that, in total, is suspected to be double the size of Texas. It is almost entirely composed of plastic. In an article in *The Independent*, one oceanographer compared the giant plastic mass to "a big animal without a leash" that occasionally "barfs" a "confetti of plastic" over pristine Hawaiian beaches.[1] Plastic floats indiscriminately throughout the world's oceans, from the polar regions to the equator, and washes up on populated beaches and uninhabited islands alike. A United Nations Environment Program report found that there were 46,000 pieces of plastic in every square mile of ocean.[2] Whether the plastic blows into the sea or is dumped there by industries, societies, or ships, it never truly goes away. It does, however, break down into smaller and smaller pieces over time. The combination of salt water and sunlight eventually wears the plastic garbage down to millions of tiny pellets no bigger than grains of sand. The plastic pieces can pick up other chemicals and pollutants before they are ingested by the fish and marine life swimming by. People catch and eat the fish, extra chemicals included. Marcus Eriksen, research director of the Algalita Marine Research Foundation, put it this way in *The Independent*: "What goes into the ocean goes into these animals and onto your dinner plate. It's that simple."

Plastic, in one of its myriad forms, is ubiquitous. In fact, it was almost by accident that Dr. Bernard Weiss, a professor of Environmental Medicine and Pediatrics at the University of Rochester School of Medicine and Dentistry, stumbled upon a startling finding connecting vinyl flooring—which is made from plastic—and autism in 2009. He wasn't looking for a vinyl flooring link, but in Sweden, where his study was conducted, standard medical questionnaires are incredibly detailed and include questions about indoor environments. The study began by looking at responses to the questionnaires for all parents of children ages 1–6 in one Swedish county in 2000 and then followed up again in 2005, asking if those children, now ages 6–8, had been assessed with autism in the intervening years. Among the topics covered was home flooring, including polyvinyl chloride or PVC flooring. "A greater proportion of children with ASD were reported to have PVC as flooring material in the child's and parent's bedroom in 2000 compared to children without ASD. Furthermore, children with ASD were reported to live in homes with more condensation on the inside of windows," an indication of poor ventilation. In the 2005 follow-up, a similar association was found. This time, PVC flooring in the parent's bedroom was "significantly associated" with autism in children along with "condensation on the windows during the winter time."[3]

In the case of PVC flooring, the suspect was a class of worrisome industrial compounds called phthalates. Phthalates soften plastic and give it flexibility, and they are found in an almost endless list of consumer products including rubber ducks and other toys, bath books, teething products, wall coverings, plastic food containers, perfumes, lotions, nail polish, varnishes and lacquers, and even pill coatings. Ingestion of phthalates can come from eating food stored in plastic containers, from babies chewing on plastic toys and teethers, from medical injections given from plastic IV bags, from drinking contaminated well water, or from breathing air containing phthalates. In the case of the Sweden study, Dr. Weiss theorizes that the phthalates were present in household dust, and were being inhaled as a result of inadequate ventilation. Until his study came out, phthalates' health effects were mostly tied to reproductive problems. The association makes sense, since the chemicals are known endocrine disruptors, or chemicals that interfere with the body's normal hormone and gland functions, blocking the action of hormones in the body, altering hormone production, or changing the chemical messages hormones are sending. These hormone activities are tied to a host of bodily functions, from metabolism to sleep to reproduction. Phthalates, disrupting this system, had been linked to the feminization of male brains, to defective development of male genitals, to lower semen quality, and to high rates of early puberty in girls. But for the first time, phthalates were also seen as a suspect in autism. "It's not the kind of thing you would publicize as the answer to autism," Dr. Weiss says, "but it certainly is a clue, that here's another chemical besides pesticides that seems to play a role in cooperating with the genetic background to produce this disability. It's one of many possible chemicals that effect brain development."[4]

Research from the Mount Sinai School of Medicine in New York has found that phthalate concentrations in pregnant women do appear to correlate with later autism-related social and behavior problems in children, "specifically poorer scores for the Orientation and Motor scales and overall Quality of Alertness, as well as more externalizing behavior problems (i.e., hyperactivity, aggressiveness) and poorer executive functioning in later childhood."[5]

About four billion pounds of just one phthalate—di-(2oethylhexyl) phthalate or DEHP—are produced in the US each year.[6] Industry spokespeople insist that they are safe, and the American Chemistry Council (ACC) has produced its own online Phthalate Information Center to counteract all the bad press. The ACC emphasizes that studies finding phthalates to be dangerous have been inconclusive, and that, in any case, "the phthalates of most concern are generally thousands of times lower than the lowest adverse effect levels for these phthalates, even in the most sensitive animal species."[7] But one of Dr. Weiss's colleagues, Dr. Shanna H. Swan at the University of Rochester, says that phthalates don't have to be present in high doses to cause serious damage. Earlier studies had discoverd that when rats were exposed to phthalates prenatally, it altered their reproductive systems.[8] Swan's research found the same held true for human boys—that prenatal pthalate exposure led to testes that didn't fully descend and shorter anogenital distance, as measured at about 16 months. The phthalate amounts in question—found in prenatal urine samples—were "below those found in one-quarter of the female population" in the US. The findings, she writes, "support the hypothesis that prenatal phthalate exposure at environmental levels can adversely affect male reproductive development in humans."[9]

At a 2011 "Greening Our Children" luncheon supporting Mount Sinai's research efforts, Dr. Swan told the seven hundred in attendance that when it comes to phthalates, "the tiniest amount—a drop in an Olympic-sized swimming pool—can make a difference during a specific window of development."[10] DEHP is found in foods packaged in plastics, including milk and fish, and in plastic tubing, including the tubing that provides life support to vulnerable infants in neonatal intensive care units. Another phthalate, dibutyl phthalate (DBP), is found in hairspray and nail polish and other dyes and lacquers, as well as the coatings of medicines. The more a mother is exposed to these phthalates, the more likely she is to have a son with less testosterone, undescended testicles, a small penis, and shorter anogenital distance, and who, more generally, "plays in a less masculine way."[11] A 2010 memo from the US Consumer Product Safety Commission assessing the health risks related to DBP found that "animal studies show an increased incidence of undescended testes, hypospadias [a birth defect in which the urethra is on the underside, rather than the end, of the penis], reproductive organ malformations, and nipple retention in males. In females, the data shows altered estrogen cyclicity and delayed maturation. The data," the paper concludes, "is sufficient to consider DBP developmentally toxic under the FHSA [Federal Hazardous Substances Act]."[12]

California was the first state to act on phthalate concerns surrounding children's health, banning the chemical from children's products beginning in 2009. Tests conducted in San Francisco leading up to the ban found that there was little uniformity—and no control—when it came to toy phthalate levels. In a toy pony, for example, one sample contained no phthalate levels, while another sample contained 40 percent.[13] Major retailers such as Walmart, Toys "R" Us, and Target, preempting public relations disasters tied to increasing concerns with phthalates, had already begun to act, voluntarily removing phthalate-containing kids' toys and teething products from shelves. But the federal Consumer Product Safety Commission, which is supposed to protect the public from unsafe products, attempted to thwart California's attempts to fully implement the ban, by allowing any phthalate-containing products made before February of 2009 to continue to be sold indefinitely. Though the agency found DBP to be "toxic" based on many animal and human health studies according to its 2010 memo, it found that "the determination of potential injury or illness cannot be concluded at this time." In the end, the courts decided. A lawsuit brought by the Natural Resources Defense Council and Public Citizen fought the exemption and won. Now, despite arguments from the ACC, children's products—specifically any toy or product that could be put in the mouth—containing more than .1 percent of phthalates are prohibited from sale across the United States.[14] Parents will no longer be forced to wonder whether the My Little Pony toy they are buying for their child is the one laden with phthalates.

Phthalates have been successfully challenged with regard to children's products, but exposure to the chemical from other sources remains widespread. And they are just one among several endocrine disruptors that have risen to the surface of the autism discussion—a list that includes PCBs, BPA, and organophosphate pesticides. "Imagine a massive experiment in which thousands of animals are exposed to hundreds of chemicals in the air, food and water," Dr. Swan told the luncheon attendees. "We are all participating in this experiment today without our consent. These are stealth chemicals . . . and there are consequences."

PCBs are stubbornly persistent in the environment, despite the fact that the country stopped manufacturing them in August of 1977. The synthetic, organic chemicals have no smell or taste, and were used as either oily liquids or nearly colorless solids to cool and lubricate electrical parts like transformers. Older buildings may still have PCB-containing fluorescent lights, electrical devices, and appliances, but most exposure today comes from the waste left behind, much of which has been improperly dumped or stored, or ineffectively burned. In 2000, at least 500 of the then nearly 1,600 current or former hazardous waste sites across the nation on the National Priorities List were found to be contaminated with dangerous levels of leaked PCBs.[15] The pastoral-looking Hudson River in New York, for instance, was contaminated beneath with more than a million pounds of PCBs dumped by two General Electric plants. Despite expensive cleanup efforts, tens of thousands of pounds of the chemicals remain, and will likely continue to remain indefinitely.[16] And PCBs don't stay where they are dumped or stored. The lightest PCBs travel and settle like little chemical messengers across the globe, evaporating from the soil and water to become airborne, and falling again wherever raindrops or snowflakes are formed, even in the Arctic. They build up in the leaves of plants and in fish and animals, and the older and higher up the food chain a creature is, the more PCBs it contains.[17] We breathe PCB-laden dust and eat meat and fish or drink milk from animals that have accumulated PCBs in their fatty tissues, and the PCBs take up residence in our bodies, too.

When levels of PCBs found in a highly exposed mother's blood or breast milk are duplicated in pregnant and nursing rats, the chemicals have been shown to cause devastating impacts on brain development. Dr. Merzenich at the University of California, San Francisco discovered that when he fed one type of PCBs to rat mothers during and following pregnancy, it damaged the rat pups' auditory cortexes, the part of the brain that processes sound. The nerve cells in this part of the brain were unable to "learn" in response to sound, and, as such, unable to develop higher language and learning ability. It's the same part of the brain that's damaged in individuals with autism.[18]

This significant damage to the animals' brains was evident after "very plausibly realistic levels of PCB intoxication,"[19] Dr. Merzenich says. In animal models the chemical could be impacting the developing young either in utero or during the course of breastfeeding as PCBs pass through the mother's milk; in any case, it left the infant animal brains in a permanently primitive state. Dr. Merzenich theorized that a child who might otherwise develop a minor impairment when exposed to PCBs could, due to genetic risk, be chemically pushed into a much more serious condition like autism.

PCBs concentrate in fatty breast milk at six times the levels they build up in regular body tissues. According to Dr. Merzenich, "In a sense the mother is concentrating these poisons and delivering them in relatively high dose levels to infants."[20] In the 1970s, when breastfeeding in the US was at an all-time low, only 24 percent of women breastfed their babies,[21] but more mothers today are choosing to breastfeed in order to access the positive health benefits of better infant growth and reduced likelihood of asthma, allergies, and type-2 diabetes. The CDC reports that 77 percent of infants born from 2005 to 2006 were breastfed. Thirty-five percent of white infants and 40 percent of Mexican American infants were breastfed six months or longer.

Like lead and mercury, PCBs have an insidious capacity to build up in the body's tissues, and these metals and chemicals interfere with the body's production of the chemical compound heme, a building block for hemoglobin, the iron-containing component of red blood cells that helps transport oxygen to, and carbon dioxide from, the body's tissues. The level of compounds called porphyrins in a person's urine can be used as a biomarker for PCB and mercury exposure, letting researchers know the level of exposure to these toxins that a person has experienced.[22] A 2010 study found that children with autism have elevated levels of porphyrins in their urine, although mercury exposure via fish consumption or dental fillings for the autistic kids and typical kids they looked at were comparable. The authors concluded that "disordered porphyrin metabolism" was "a salient characteristic of autism," though this condition did not appear to be related to past mercury exposure.[23] But another 2010 study found a direct relationship between urinary porphyrin levels indicating levels of mercury toxicity and scores on a series of measurements that define autism symptoms including speech and language, sociability, and sensory and cognitive awareness. The greater the levels of "urinary porphyrin biomarkers of mercury toxicity" the greater the magnitude of autistic behaviors in the categories measured.[24]

Besides phthalates and PCBs, nearly everyone in the US ingests the chemical BPA on a regular, if not daily, basis. An industrial chemical, BPA is used to make shatterproof or polycarbonate plastic for products like water bottles, baby bottles, food storage containers, plastic dinnerware, the lenses of glasses, milk containers, and dental sealants. It coats cash register receipts, and it also lines most canned food in the US. The process of making these plastic components is imperfect; BPA molecules are linked together to form the plastic, but some remain unlinked. These rogue molecules are absorbed into food supplies during the process of storing, preparing, eating, and drinking. Certain foods are particularly prone to BPA leaching from the lining of cans, like tomatoes and infant formula. In 2007, the Environmental Working Group rounded up a collection of common canned foods from major chain grocery stores in Atlanta, Georgia, Oakland, California, and Clinton, Connecticut, including soda, canned tuna, peaches and pineapples, green beans, corn, and tomato and chicken noodle soups, and sent them to a lab for testing. The selection included twenty-seven national brands and three store brands. Some 57 percent of all cans contained detectable levels of BPA, but certain foods had particularly worrisome levels. The foods with the highest BPA content were those often used to feed infants and toddlers: liquid infant formula, chicken soup, and ravioli. The concentrations of BPA in these foods meant that in just one to three servings, a woman or child would be exposed to levels of BPA 200 times more than the government's safety level.[25] A 2009 testing of canned food by *Consumer Reports* found that the chemicals were present even in items labeled organic and "BPA-free."[26] In the US, nearly all of us have measurable amounts of BPA in our urine, according to tests done by the CDC.[27]

As a chemical, BPA's popularity is almost unrivalled. Produced at a rate of more than 8 billion pounds per year,[28] it is ubiquitous in commerce and one of the most common industrial waste products. One million pounds per year are released into the environment, according to the EPA; it contaminates the air and water supplies and settles in household dust.[29] The chemical was initially designed in 1891 as a synthetic estrogen to mimic the sex hormone estradiol, produced in women's ovaries. But BPA was considered a weak estrogen, so it found limited use as a hormone treatment. In the 1950s, BPA had a resurgence as the foundation for shatterproof polycarbonate plastic used for bottles and dishware, and as the epoxy resin lining for food cans. With its rise in popularity came new government tests in the 1970s to ensure that increased human exposure was safe. There were concerns, perhaps not surprisingly, that the synthetic hormone could disrupt reproductive development, particularly in males, and lead to cancers related to the reproductive system, like breast and prostate cancer.[30] Those concerns were well founded; according to studies, adverse effects from BPA could happen at extremely low doses, far below exposures experienced by adults, developing fetuses, and many fish and other organisms in the natural world. In the late 1990s Frederick vom Saal, curators professor of biological sciences at the University of Missouri, found that just 50 femtograms—or .05 trillionths of a gram—of a synthetic hormone like BPA in a milliliter of blood caused profound changes in an animal's development. The list of these impacts was long and unsettling. In an interview with the PBS show *Frontline* conducted just after the results were released, vom Saal said, "We see changes in the functioning of the prostate. We see dramatic change in the sprouting of glands within the fetal prostate. We see changes in testicular sperm production. We see changes in the structure of the endocrine control region in the brain, which is accompanied by changes in sex behavior, aggression, the way these animals behave towards infants, their whole social interaction, the way they age, the time that they enter puberty, the age at which they cease reproduction. It changes their entire life history, and these changes are capable of occurring at very low levels of hormones."[31]

One of the basic reasons BPA was originally deemed safe was the widely held belief among the science community that food was the main route of exposure, and that BPA was excreted quickly. In a 2009 study by the University of Rochester Medical Center that challenged this assumption, researchers write that BPA exposure "is thought to be almost entirely from food." They add that "in human adults, BPA is generally described as raidly metabolized, with elimination thought to be virtually complete within 24 hours of exposure." Following that logic, researchers expected that people's BPA levels would decrease by half every five hours during fasting. Instead, according to the study, even after people fasted for twenty-four hours, levels of BPA in their bodies remained stubbornly high. That led researchers to conclude that additional exposure was happening somewhere else—that BPA was present in household dust or tap water, for example—or that the chemical was taking up residence in fat tissues where it would be released more slowly. Dr. Swan and the other researchers posited that more investigation was necessary to "search for important nonfood sources."[32]

One such source is cash register receipts. Studies commissioned by the Environmental Working Group found BPA in amounts ranging from .8 to nearly 3 percent pure BPA by weight on receipts from major retailers and outlets like McDonald's, CVS, KFC, Whole Foods, Walmart, Safeway, and the US Postal Service. The chemical transfers easily to and is capable of penetrating the skin, potentially entering the bloodstream directly; it can also be ingested when BPA-tainted fingers enter the mouth.[33]

BPA has been found in all the fluids, tissues, and blood supplies that provide nourishment to a fetus: pregnant women's blood, amniotic fluid, placental tissue, and umbilical cord blood. The chemical has also been detected in breast milk. And infants—at least infant rats—appear less able to metabolize BPA than adult animals, so higher concentrations of the chemical are circulating freely in their blood.[34] Infant bodies can't tell the difference between BPA and the sex hormone estradiol, and the presence of this false hormone alters their development from the earliest stages, changing the way cells grow, giving rise to larger prostates, and increasing the hormone that puts a person at risk for breast cancer, among other effects. Rat cells and human cells respond to such hormones nearly identically. According to vom Saal, the impacts of BPA on the way an infant's organs develop during critical periods of development are permanent and irreversible. "Once you change the development of an organ there is no way to undo that effect," he told *Frontline*. "It's a life sentence—that's a lifetime consequence. Medical science can't undo the development of organs." Following his warnings, two studies tried to replicate vom Saal's findings with low doses of BPA, but did not reach the same results. But both of these studies were funded by an industry group, the European Chemical Industry Council, and one of them was actually performed by BPA producers.[35]

In subsequent years, vom Saal has become increasingly outspoken about the risks posed by BPA and the failure of the federal government to take protective action. BPA, along with 61,000 other chemicals, was grandfathered in under the Toxic Substances Control Act (TSCA) of 1976, meaning they were exempt from testing for environmental or human health effects. Despite the fact that in January 2010 the FDA reversed its position on BPA and expressed concerns about its health impacts, saying that "recent studies provide reason for some concern about the potential effects of BPA on the brain, behavior, and prostate gland of fetuses, infants and children,"[36] the agency has still been unable to regulate the chemical because of its exemption status under TSCA. To put it simply, the federal agency charged with protecting consumers' health has publicly declared that BPA is dangerous, but is powerless to regulate it. Efforts at the Congressional level led by California Democratic Senator Dianne Feinstein to ban BPA from children's bottles and sippy cups were stymied by obstructions from the American Chemical Council in November 2010, and vom Saal has said that in his early days of researching BPA he was personally threatened by chemical manufacturers. The researcher told the online publication *Yale Environment 360* in November 2010 that "changing the rules that we operate by, if we had a compliant industry, would take five to 10 years. And this is one extremely non-compliant industry. [BPA is] almost a $10 billion-a-year product. You know, people don't give up that kind of money."[37]

BPA's potential link to autism is less clear, but it is a subject of growing concern. A December 2010 study conducted by researchers from the Mount Sinai School of Medicine in New York connected both phthalates and BPA with childhood social impairments associated with autism, including difficulties in communication and recognizing and responding to social cues. They looked at 404 women who had delivered at Mount Sinai Hospital between May 1998 and July 2002, primarily from the largely minority urban community of East Harlem, New York. They measured the mothers' urine samples for phthalates and BPA during the third trimester, then invited the women to return for follow-up visits when their children were between four and nine years old. Not all did, of course—in fact, just 137 women returned for later testing—but among those that did there was a clear association between higher levels of phthalates and BPA in the moms' third trimester urine and children scoring lower on the Social Responsiveness Scale (SRS) between the ages of 7 and 9, a "rating scale of social behaviors characteristic of autism spectrum and related disorders."[38] The association was clearer between phthalates and later social difficulties, in part because BPA was more diluted in urine samples. Nonetheless, the study found that, "In unadjusted models, we found a positive correlation of . . . phthalate . . . and BPA level with total SRS. Positive correlations reflect poorer SRS scores with increasing BPA and phthalate metabolite concentrations." In adjusted models, the correlation between BPA and poor SRS scores was not evident, although the correlation between phthalate exposure and lower SRS scores remained.[39] It was the first study to connect "social behavior in school-aged children in relation to prenatal exposure to BPA and phthalates," and it indicates that endocrine-disrupting industrial chemicals can contribute to problems in brain development and functioning causing social impairments that have lifetime implications.[40]

BPA has also been found to significantly impact the genetic process of DNA methylation, in which the cells of the body, beginning with the same genetic blueprint, differentiate into liver cells, heart cells, and brain cells. As is discussed in the introduction, scientists now think this process does not just happen in the early stages of life, but continues into old age, with changes happening to our cells in response to environmental stressors and chemicals. Dr. Randy Jirtle, the director of the epigenetics and imprinting laboratory at Duke University, has described that interaction as akin to the way computer software guides the way the computer hardware works. The epigenomes, in charge of the genes, determine precisely how those genes—and subsequently, cells and organs—will ultimately function. Dr. Jirtle tested the epigenetic impacts of BPA on mice with identical DNA by introducing the chemical during pregnancy. Mice exposed to BPA during pregnancy gave birth to baby mice that had unusual, lemon-yellow fur, and, in many cases, developed obesity, diabetes, and cancer as adults. Mice with the same DNA that were not exposed developed to normal size, had typical brown coats, and were not prone to the same diseases. In the BPA-exposed mice, the chemical reduced the DNA methylation process, preventing a gene known as the agouti gene from being turned off, leaving the animals vulnerable to dangerous diseases. When the same pregnant mice were fed a diet that included folic acid and vitamin B-12, supplements that increase cells' methylation, these risk factors were greatly reduced.[41]

In a related article, researcher Jill Adams wrote,

When gene expression goes awry during development, as in bisphenol-exposed mouse pups, the consequences can cause changes in adult mice that were not seen at birth. This phenomenon, called fetal programming, may play a role in many health conditions, including heart disease, diabetes, obesity, and cancer. The yellow agouti mouse is a great animal model for studies in epigenetics and fetal programming. Recently, it has also been used to show that dietary factors can prevent the agouti gene from being turned on. More specifically, not only did Jirtle's group find an increased risk of disease with maternal chemical exposure in mice, but they also noted that certain nutrients [folic acid and B-12] were protective. . . . In addition, a constituent of soy products called genistein prevented an increased number of unhealthy offspring. Whether a similar diet might reverse epigenetic effects once they appear, however, is unknown and awaits experimental testing. Despite such uncertainties, this epigenetic mechanism clearly demonstrates how profoundly environment can affect gene expression and phenotype in a long-lasting way.[42]

Whether this methylation process's alteration by BPA or other environmental exposures is a risk factor for autism is not yet clear, but there's increasing evidence that methylation plays a role in the disorder. As is discussed in Chapter 5, some research has zeroed in on the importance of the hormone oxytocin—the "social hormone" that promotes early mother-infant bonding and social interaction as a baby begins to navigate his or her world. A study at Duke University conducted by Dr. Simon Gregory found that in individuals with autism, a gene tied to production of oxytocin was more methylated, which could be responsible for lowering a person's sensitivity to the hormone, resulting in the social isolation that is a hallmark of autism. And researchers are only beginning to understand the effect of DNA methylation on the human body's 20,000 to 25,000 genes. "DNA methylation," says Dr.

Shuk-mei Ho at the University of Cincinnati, "acts as a permanent lock for a gene, turning off a gene for a long time."[43] The Human Epigenome Project, which has set out to identify and catalog all the ways DNA methylation works in the body's tissues, reports that DNA methylation is thought to play a role in all human diseases and "constitutes the main and so far missing link between genetics, disease and the environment."[44]

Jill James's research has found that both parents of children with autism and the children themselves have difficulties related to methylation on the same gene. She also found that they had lower-than-normal levels of the antioxidant glutathione and less "detoxification capacity."[45] This combination of traits combines to form a metabolic imbalance, altering the way the body breaks food down into glucose, a sugar that's the body's basic source of energy. When glucose travels through the bloodstream to the pancreas, the gland organ in our digestive systems, it triggers the pancreas to release the hormone insulin. Insulin tells the body's tissues whether to convert the glucose to energy or store it as fat. When this system is imbalanced, as James has found among children with autism and their parents, their bodies are less able to convert glucose, which may cause the build-up of fats at unhealthy levels. Their bodies are similarly overwhelmed with toxins, as they are unable to protect cells from damage by removing toxic intruders, such as chemicals. These genetic traits, she found, appear to be hereditary, and may, in fact, be epigenetic in nature. At present, James reports, it is unclear whether the metabolic abnormalities related to autism are genetically based or are triggered by unhealthy diets or chronic environmental exposures.

The epigenome—the "ghost in our genes," or hidden programmer—exists, researchers believe, to help bodies adapt to changes in the environment, to give us advantages over time. Unfortunately, as Dr. Ho explains, the onslaught of chemicals in our natural world, as well as our own bad habits like smoking and even our ability to move between countries and continents, has thrown this system off, putting us at a disadvantage.

"During development," Dr. Ho says, "some tissue or organs will take a few days to become fully differentiated, others will take many weeks. And others will take many months. For example, brains and neurons will take years, up to 20 or 25 years. So during this whole period of differentiation when the tissue or organ is not fully mature, there are still many opportunities for the environment to interact, to give information to the cell, and the cell could modify and change the epigenome in a way to be adaptive." If these early adaptive changes within the cells match the body's demands later in life, the result is a healthy life. If they don't, the result is an increase in disease, whether cancer, obesity, or autism. Many environmental factors are contributing to this mismatch between our genetic programming and later life demands, from lifestyle choices like smoking and alcohol consumption, to diets high in fatty foods, to high levels of stress, to exposure to thousands of chemicals—all of which have no adaptive advantage. And these epigenetic changes, brought on by any number of choices or exposures, can be passed on to children and grandchildren.

Such passing on of traits was discovered inadvertently when researchers looked at the long-term effects of the Dutch famine known as "Hunger Winter" in Holland between 1944 and 1945, the final year of World War II. The Nazis, nearing the end of a losing battle with Allied forces, imposed a punishing blockade on food and fuel supplies that left much of Holland to starve, and forced the population to consume everything from animal blood to tulip bulbs to survive. During the seven months that the blockade went on, adults were eating just four hundred to eight hundred calories a day (a daily ration consisted of a couple slices of bread, two potatoes, and a sugar beet), less than a quarter of their recommended intake. It was the timing of the famine during gestation that played the greatest role in infants developing diseases in adulthood. Mothers who were subjected to a starvation diet during the first trimester of their pregnancies gave birth to infants who later "experienced elevated rates of obesity, altered lipid profiles, and cardiovascular disease" as adults.[46]

The fact that drastic changes in lifestyle and environmental exposures to chemicals can change the programming of genes and alter a person's likelihood for disease could help unlock other mysteries related to autism, such as why certain immigrant populations develop an increased risk when they relocate, as happened with the Somali families in Sweden whose children were three to four times as likely to have autism as children in nonimmigrant families.[47] A similar phenomenon was seen in Minnesota, where there were a significantly higher number of Somali children enrolled in the state's ASD programs.[48] It's possible that the sudden changes in diet, climate, environmental exposures, and the stress associated with relocation for these immigrants may have played a role in altering their children's genetic programming, making them more susceptible to autism.

If a chemical—or combination of chemicals—had an epigenetic impact that could be passed from generation to generation, it would also go a long way in explaining why autism cases continue to increase with each passing year. While the link between BPA and autism is still being established, other endocrine disruptors introduced during fetal development have been shown to give rise to a long list of diseases, not just in the first generation, but into the fourth generation. Dr. Michael Skinner, a principal investigator in the School of Biological Sciences at Washington State University, found that when rats were exposed to one fungicide called vinclozolin, used primarily today to control diseases on wine grapes and on golf course turf, it induced diseases into subsequent generations of rats, including "prostate disease, kidney disease, immune system abnormalities, testis abnormalities, and tumor development." The incidences of these diseases was "high and consistent across all generations" and appeared "to be due in part to epigenetic alterations."[49] Since 2000 the EPA has revoked most use of vinclozolin on crops due to its health impacts on children, but use of vinclozolin was allowed for another three years before it was fully phased out, so the chemical continued to contaminate meat and dairy products; tomatoes, plums, grapes, and strawberries; and water supplies. At low doses in rats, exposure to vinclozolin resulted in decreased prostate size and shorter anogenital distance. At higher doses, it resulted in deformed sex organs, including undescended testes and vaginal pouches as well as testicular tumors. It may also, the agency reports, affect the development and functioning of the neuroendocrine system—the way the nervous system and the endocrine system interact—which would impact the development and functioning of the brain.[50] And the link between such devastating health effects in rats and humans is well established. The EPA notes that the androgen receptor in rats that is impacted by vinclozolin is widely conserved across species lines, so that these same impacts "would be expected in humans."[51]

The four hundred-mile stretch known as the Central Valley in California is America's agricultural Mecca. The flat, fertile farmland there supplies one-quarter of the food consumed in the US. But the need for productive yields has also meant the region is home to a concentrated level of chemicals that may have given rise to higher autism rates for those families living close by. Cotton and other crops in the Central Valley were routinely sprayed with older, dangerous pesticides known as organochlorines, pesticides that persist both in the environment and peoples' bodies. The first widespread organochlorine to gain public attention was DDT, used for three decades to combat pests in fields, forests, and backyards. It was known as a "miracle" pesticide for its effectiveness, and at its height in 1962, the US Department of Health and Human Services reports that more than one hundred eighty million pounds of DDT were produced in the US for agricultural use across the country.[52]

In 1945, when nature writer and former marine biologist Rachel Carson first proposed writing about DDT's dangerous after-effects on the natural world for *Reader's Digest*, the magazine rejected her proposal. But Carson spent years gathering research on the topic—research that would later take shape as *Silent Spring*, the story of one dangerous chemical run amok. *Silent Spring* details how DDT builds up in the body fat of animals and is passed up the food chain; how it kills insects indiscriminately; and how it persists in the environment, contaminating food supplies, birds, and animals across the world. In the book's most famous chapter, "A Fable for Tomorrow," Carson imagines a once-idyllic, fictional town struck silent by "a shadow of death." In this altered place, where chicks failed to hatch and bees stopped pollinating fruits and streams held no fish, she writes: "the doctors had become more and more puzzled by new kinds of sickness appearing among their patients. There had been several sudden and unexplained deaths, not only among adults but even among children, who would be stricken suddenly while at play and die within a few hours." She wrote with eloquence and haunting precision about the impact of chemicals so widely applied and so rarely questioned, including the pesticides, the "nonselective chemicals that have the power to kill every insect, the 'good' and the 'bad,' to still the song of birds and the leaping of fish in the streams, to coat the leaves with a deadly film, and to linger on in soil—all this though the intended target may be only a few weeds or insects." Carson asked, pointedly: "Can anyone believe it is possible to lay down such a barrage of poisons on the surface of the earth without making it unfit for all life? They should not be called 'insecticides,' but 'biocides.'"[53]

Her work spurred national indignation at our thoughtless chemical assault, helping to launch the modern environmental movement. It brought the Kennedy administration to study the impact of DDT, and it led the Nixon administration to establish the EPA, tasked with overseeing "air pollution, water pollution and solid wastes as different forms of a single problem."[54] Finally, eight years after Carson's death and ten years after the EPA was formed, DDT was banned by that very agency when it was discovered that exposure could lead to nervous system problems, including tremors and seizures, as well as increasing the risk for giving birth prematurely and reducing a mother's ability to produce milk. In its 1972 decision, the EPA wrote that "the continued massive use of DDT posed unacceptable risks to the environment and potential harm to human health."[55]

But Carson rightly saw that DDT's once liberal application would remain the nation's toxic legacy to endure. The chemical, having accumulated over thirty years of widespread application in soil, plants, and the fatty tissues of fish, birds, and other animals, has never gone away. The EPA has discovered DDT and similar compounds in at least 441 of the nation's current National Priorities List sites.[56]

Now other pesticides in the same class as DDT have been tied to autism. In the Central Valley, researchers found that the closer pregnant mothers lived to fields growing cotton, fruit, vegetables, beans, and other crops sprayed with endosulfan and dicofol, the more likely they were to give birth to children with autism. They found 465 children with autism born across nineteen counties between Sacramento and the San Joaquin River valleys between 1996 and 1998. Researchers noted that "ASD risk increased with the poundage of organochlorine applied and decreased with distance from field sites."[57] Because the study was small, it was deemed another cautionary tale, rather than a definitive answer. The study's lead author, Eric M. Roberts, could only report, "It's not something someone's offering as an answer. It's just something to keep in mind."[58]

ADHD also increases in likelihood the closer pregnant mothers live to pesticide-sprayed fields. It is now thought that both autism and ADHD share a "risk gene." Of the body's 20,000 to 25,000 genes, researchers in 2002 zeroed in on one region of about 100 to 150 genes underlying both autism and ADHD called chromosome 16.[59] If the two disorders share a genetic basis, then it's possible that environmental exposures to some combination of chemicals could be the missing link, pushing a susceptible child to one side or the other during pregnancy. When researchers studied children born to Mexican American women in the Salinas Valley, a region where more than one million pounds of herbicides, fungicides, and pesticides are applied to crops each year,[60] they found that the higher the concentrations of organophosphate metabolites in pregnant women's urine, the more likely they were to have young children with "attention problems and poorer attention scores." The association was stronger at five years than three years and "generally stronger in boys."[61]

Organophosphate pesticides are just as toxic as organochlorines like DDT, but since they are less chemically stable and so less likely to accumulate, they have not been banned for use on crops. Both types of pesticides have been shown to impact infants who are exposed prenatally, affecting their early reflex abilities, a critical marker of proper brain development. Organophosphate pesticides disrupt the formation of neurotransmitters necessary for proper brain development, including a person's ability to pay attention and remember. And children and developing infants "are more vulnerable to organophosphate exposure than adults because of lower levels of acetylcholinesterase, which detoxifies these pesticides," a related report notes. The study's senior author, Brenda Eskenazi, a professor at UC Berkeley, says that risks can be minimized by thoroughly washing fruits and vegetables. "It's known that food is a significant source of pesticide exposure among the general population," she said. "I would recommend thoroughly washing fruits and vegetables before eating them, especially if you're pregnant."[62]

Pesticides used inside the home to combat roaches, ticks, fleas, and other pests can have lasting consequences, too. Researchers in California asked hundreds of mothers who have children with autism a series of questions about their household habits, including their use of insecticides against fleas or ants, their use of weed killers, and their use of flea-killing pet shampoos. The latter product is the one that stood out; mothers of children with autism were twice as likely as mothers of typical children to report having used pet shampoos or sprays for fleas or ticks during pregnancy, particularly during the second trimester.[63] These common pest-control products contain an insecticide that's far less toxic than those sprayed across crops. Their flea- and tick-killing properties come from pyrethrin, a substance derived from chrysanthemum flowers that works as an immediate nerve poison to insects. For humans, there is thought to be little danger associated with pyrethrin except possible allergic reactions, such as coughing, wheezing, or rashes. But rats that have been fed high doses of pyrethrin have shown difficult or rapid breathing, as well as tremors, aggression, increased sensitivity, and twitching. Particularly worrisome in relation to autism is the way pyrethrins act on fetal brains in rodents, compromising the blood-brain barrier, the four hundred miles of narrow capillaries that protect the brain by barring dangerous chemicals from entry. And pyrethrins can linger in the home, particularly on pet hairs, increasing human exposure.[64]

Inner city residents, meanwhile, were at one time commonly exposed to a pesticide called chlorpyrifos (CPF), used to control cockroaches. The pesticide was found to directly impact brain and motor development in kids, and the EPA banned it from residential use beginning in 2001.[65] The three-year study from Columbia University initiated in 1997 that made the connection focused on New York City residents, many of whom sprayed or otherwise treated their homes for cockroaches on a weekly basis. In fact, the study found "detectable levels of chlorpyrifos . . . in 99.7% of personal air samples and 100% of indoor air samples from stationary residential monitors for a sample of pregnant women."[66] Detected in 64 to 70 percent of blood samples from pregnant women and newborns, the chemical levels correlated strongly between mother and child, indicating that the pesticide easily crosses the placenta. Higher chlorpyrifos levels in children also directly correlated with lower birth weights and lengths, but what researchers were particularly interested in were the long-term impacts of the early pesticide exposure on learning and behavior that may not be evident until the preschool years.

The study focused on children born to black and Dominican New York City residents between 1998 and 2002. The umbilical cord blood was tested for chlorpyrifos levels at birth. They were given developmental assessment tests at twelve, twenty-four, and thirty-six months. There were 536 active participants among the women (all nonsmoking), and 189 children who were able to be measured at all three points. After researchers controlled for other factors related to the home environment, lead exposure, and a mother's education level, they found a clear association between pesticide exposure and developmental delay. The group who scored the lowest on the Bayley Scales of Infant Development II at age three was the group with the highest exposure levels to the cockroach-killing pesticide. The study reports that "children exposed to high levels of chlorpyrifos scored lower, on average, on 5 of the 6 age-specific tests than did children exposed to lower levels." These highly exposed children were also much more likely to have more serious developmental problems, including attention problems, ADHD, or PDD. Among the three-year-olds studied, 4.7 percent overall had PDD problems, compared to 8.5 percent of those in the high-exposure group. ADHD affected 3.9 percent of kids overall, and 10.6 percent of those who had been highly exposed. Chlorpyrifos exposure had a damaging effect not just on brain and behavior development, but "adverse cognitive and psychomotor effects increased over time," and were more apt to lead a child to lifelong learning problems via ADHD or PDD.[67]

Despite the ban on residential use, chlorpyrifos—manufactured by the Dow Chemical Company under the names Dursban and Lorsban—remains one of the most common organophosphate insecticides applied on crops worldwide. The EPA reports that 10 million pounds of chlorpyrifos are applied to US crops each year, including corn (for which 5.5 million pounds of the pesticide is used annually), citrus plants, alfalfa, and peanuts. The pesticide is also widely applied to golf courses and used as a wood treatment. Residues remain on nonorganic fruits and vegetables.

Those living near or working on massive farms are at the greatest risk for exposure, but pesticides can be ingested in smaller amounts by eating the tainted fruits and vegetables grown on these fields. In one study conducted at the University of Washington, children who ate conventional diets were switched to an organic-only diet of fresh fruits, vegetables, juices, and packaged items like pasta, cereal, and chips, for five days. Urinary pesticide levels were six times higher before the switch to organic foods, and they dropped significantly to nondetectable levels, often within twenty-four hours, once the organic diets were instituted.[68]

The EPA writes that "dietary exposures from eating food crops treated with chlorpyrifos are below the level of concern for the entire US population, including infants and children."[69] But Amy Marks, the lead author of the study on ADHD with the University of California Berkeley's School of Public Health, said in a statement: "Given that these compounds are designed to attack the nervous system of organisms, there is reason to be cautious, especially in situations where exposure may coincide with critical periods of fetal and child development."[70]

Despite public concern over chemicals, it has been difficult to summon the political will to overhaul the nation's chemical regulation and initiate a move toward safer chemicals. After President Obama was elected, the Rachel Carson Council, Inc. sent him an open letter remarking that the chemical onslaught has seriously worsened since Carson's time. "The numbers and amounts of other potentially toxic chemicals in widely-used, commercial products, including plastics, non-stick cookware, and flame retardant fabrics have greatly increased. We are becoming more aware every day that these chemicals, whether considered toxic or perceived as 'safe,' are present as mixtures in the environment and in our bodies. Concurrent exposures to these agents pose new and largely unresearched, potential hazards," the letter read. The council called on the president to initiate a new era of protection, led by the precautionary principle—the idea that we should "first do no harm"—by expanding risk assessments, increasing regulation of hazardous chemicals and disclosure of chemical ingredients, and conducting field trials. The council focused on the danger posed by chemical mixtures, the most likely cause for rising autism rates from chemical exposures. "Since Carson's day," the council wrote, "we have recognized that lack of data does not necessarily mean lack of harm."[71]

In 2009, Connecticut became the first state in the nation to ban BPA from baby products, and the ban took effect in 2011.[72] That was just the beginning. Nearly forty similar measures seeking to regulate BPA—in children's products or across all food and beverage containers—were proposed across nineteen states in 2009. Chicago was the first city to pass a BPA ban, and Suffolk County, New York, was the first locality. A ban was passed in Minnesota prohibiting BPA from children's products, and bans were enacted in Maryland, Wisconsin, Washington, Vermont, and New York. In California, despite the chemical industry spending a reported $5 million to defeat the measure,[73] a bill banning BPA in children's products like sippy cups, bottles, infant formula, and baby food called the Toxin-Free Infants and Toddlers Act was signed into law in October 2011, to go into effect in 2013.[74] Also in June 2011, Connecticut became the first state to ban BPA on cash register receipts, which will be instituted July 1, 2015, unless the EPA enacts its own ban first.[75] As mentioned, major retailers took preemptive action before these bans, deciding that there was enough consumer concern to warrant removing BPA-containing baby and infant products from their store shelves voluntarily. Walmart announced it would stop stocking BPA-containing baby bottles and feeding products. Toys "R" Us followed, making plans to phase the products out of its toy stores and Babies "R" Us stores. Under pressure from attorneys general from Connecticut, New Jersey, and Delaware, the US's six major bottle manufacturers—Avent, Disney First Years, Gerber, Dr. Brown, Playtex, and Evenflow—all agreed to stop making baby bottles containing BPA.[76] Even one manufacturer of BPA, the gas and chemical company Sunoco, now refuses to sell the chemical to companies that produce food and water containers for children under age three because of concerns about its safety to children's health.[77]

In the swelling wave of concern surrounding BPA's health impacts on infants and children, all that remained was a ban at the federal level. That measure was introduced by California Senator Dianne Feinstein in 2010 as an amendment to the Food Safety and Modernization Act. But the measure was defeated before the act went to vote in the Senate over fears that the bill wouldn't pass otherwise. "The very same lobbying group that opposed legislation banning phthalates from children's toys made a last-minute push to scuttle the chances for a reasonable compromise, and Republicans bowed to pressure from the chemical industry," Sen. Feinstein later wrote on *Huffington Post*. "It is regretful that lobbyists for the American Chemistry Council, spending millions of dollars, lined up against a reasonable compromise. And it's maddening that BPA-laden baby bottles will remain on the shelves as a 'safe' product."[78] She encouraged concerned parents, in lieu of stringent federal regulation, to vote with their dollars instead.

The struggle—and ultimate failure—to ban just one chemical of concern at the federal level foreshadowed the enormous difficulty of passing any meaningful comprehensive reform. As stated, it has long been known that the existing TSCA of 1974 offers weak protection to the public in regards to chemical safety. Despite the general policies of requiring data as to the environmental and public health safety of chemicals, authorizing the EPA to regulate dangerous chemicals, and taking action when such safety regulations are violated, TSCA has been designed with an elephant-sized loophole. By its own admission, the EPA writes that "Certain substances are generally excluded from TSCA, including, among others, food, drugs, cosmetics, and pesticides."[79] Most problematically, TSCA's testing rules excluded sixty-one thousand chemicals, including formaldehyde, benzene, mercury, cyanide, benzoic acid, methane, aluminum, flourene (created when coal, gas, and garbage are burned), ammonia, and sulfuric acid, that existed when it was first enacted. Since that time, less than two hundred of these chemicals have been tested for human safety. The majority of the chemicals we are regularly exposed to through the products we use, the water we drink, and the food we eat have never been tested as to their health impacts on infants, children, developing fetuses, or even adults. The agency has effectively backed itself into a legislative corner. In order for the EPA to require new tests on any of these chemicals, it must first prove that the chemical presents a serious danger to human health or the environment. Since there is little to no such safety data in existence, it has a hard time making that case.[80]

The closest the US has come to overhauling TSCA was in 2010, when separate but similar bills were introduced in the US Senate and House: the Safe Chemicals Act and the Toxic Chemicals Safety Act. Either measure, if passed, would have closed the open-door policy toward chemicals and replaced it with a new, precautionary approach. The Safe Chemicals Act, for instance, framed our modern-day understanding of the impacts and health dangers associated with untested chemicals used so freely in commerce. It addressed the accumulation of chemicals like PCBs in the natural environment—including remote Arctic regions—and the build-up of chemical concentrations inside people, as is now shown through biomonitoring studies done by government agencies and advocacy organizations like Environmental Working Group. It expressed particular concern with the way these chemicals—even in small doses—are now known to impact developing infants and children, particularly during critical windows of development, and how they have been implicated in a growing number of diseases and disorders on the rise. What's more, the bill envisioned a future where new, safer chemicals—in a movement known as green chemistry—would replace our current outdated and unsafe chemical manufacturing. "Our plastics, by and large, are petroleum-based," said Dr. Swan at the "Greening Our Children" luncheon. "They don't have to be. There are crop-based alternatives. Ford made a car from hemp. And these [green] chemicals are not persistent—they leave bodies in a couple of hours, or, at most, a couple of days."[81] The Safe Chemicals Act foresaw new jobs, and new competitive global products, that were finally in step with the safety-first consumer regulations being adopted worldwide. All chemicals, under the act, would have had to be reviewed for human health and environmental safety, with preference given to those considered high priority. Those deemed unsafe would be restricted, and would need to be replaced by safer alternatives.

But all the extensive publicity, letter-writing campaigns to senators and representatives, EPA support, and leading scientists and researchers speaking out in favor could not match the collective weight of the $674 billion chemical industry. Both bills died before reaching a vote—even under a Democratic majority in Congress. The lobbying dollars paid off; the chemical industry spent more than $40 million on lobbying efforts in the first six months of 2010, paving the way for the bills' defeat.[82] Undaunted, the Safe Chemicals Act of 2011 was reintroduced by Sen. Frank Lautenberg (D-NJ) the following year, this time with a growing coalition of support, including a major push by the group Safer Chemicals, Healthy Families, which has enlisted the high-profile support of actress Jessica Alba. But each year such bills are reintroduced, of course, the dollars to defeat them return. And as one investigative report on the undermining of chemical reform legislation noted, it's not just money that's keeping senators and representatives from supporting these acts, its political preservation. "It's a rare congressional district that doesn't have a chemical company, processing plant, or major purveyor of consumer goods," Sheila Kaplan writes for *Politics Daily*, "a point made more than once during the negotiations, and which helped keep some Democrats from signing onto the bill."[83] Most disheartening is that, as Dr. Swan noted, safer alternatives to existing harmful chemicals exist and have successfully replaced their dangerous counterparts in other countries. In Japan, can manufacturers voluntarily began replacing canned food and drink linings with a PET film or paint coating that dramatically reduced the BPA being ingested, as indicated by blood samples.[84] The European Union's Registration, Evaluation, Authorisation and Restriction of Chemical substances (REACH) regulation, passed in 2007, will accomplish many of the goals set out by the so-far failed chemical reform bills in the US. It requires chemical manufacturers to prove the safety of their products and to register them in a central database, and where such safety standards are not met, it requires companies to replace dangerous chemicals with safer alternatives. The requirements are being phased in and are scheduled to be fully implemented in 2018. The REACH law responds to nearly identical chemical-based health and environmental concerns being faced in the US, with some one hundred thousand "existing" chemicals that had been grandfathered in prior to 1981 allowed to persist in commerce with little regulatory oversight or risk assessment. As with the proposed US laws, REACH forces all chemicals to begin at the same starting point. Whether new or existing, manufacturers have to prove that the chemicals they are making are safe before they are cleared to produce and sell them. And by centralizing information related to all chemical manufacturing, the EU is ushering in a new era of transparency, where the public can easily track the safety of such chemicals for themselves.[85]

Phthalates have been banned in Europe since 2005,[86] as they are now in the US. Europe banned formaldehyde-containing wood products years ago because the off-gassing chemical has been linked to cancer and respiratory problems, and in 2010, Obama limited the amount of formaldehyde in China-sourced wood products, like cabinets, furniture, and other products constructed from particle board.[87] But these small victories in the US have been overshadowed by lax regulations that have turned the US into a de facto dumping ground for the chemical-laden goods that Japan, Canada, and countries across Europe have banned from sale.[88] A hair treatment known as "Brazilian Blowout" touted for fighting frizz contains formaldehyde levels high enough to cause some women to lose serious amounts of hair, but it remains legal in the US. Stylists who administer it, meanwhile, complain of chest pains and sore throats. The Oregon Occupational Safety and Health Division found that formaldehyde levels in one Brazilian Blowout product labeled "formaldehyde free," ranged from 7 to 12 percent; while banned in Canada, the hair treatment is protected in the US, and the manufacturer is not even obligated to disclose its harmful ingredients. Other toxins in cosmetics permitted in US shampoos, lotions, cosmetics, perfumes, and deodorants paint a similar disturbing picture. Whereas the European Union Cosmetics Directive has banned 1,100 chemicals with known harmful health impacts from personal care products, according to one 2011 investigative report in *Earth Island Journal*, the FDA only bans or restricts eleven of those chemicals. Toxic additives that have been banned in European products but are routinely added to US cosmetic products include petroleum byproducts used in baby shampoos and bubble baths that cause cancer in animal studies; parabens in deodorants and lotions, which can act as hormone-mimicking endocrine disruptors; and lead and lead acetate, a dangerous metal tied to neurological impairments at which no level of exposure is considered safe, commonly used in lipstick and men's hair coloring products.[89]

The antibacterial chemical triclosan—an endocrine disruptor found in 75 percent of liquid soaps, 29 percent of bar soaps, cosmetics, toothpastes, deodorants, socks, shoes, cutting boards, and baby products, also poses a danger as it washes down the drain, contaminating the nation's rivers, lakes, and drinking water. The US Geological Survey (USGS) has found detectable triclosan levels in 60 percent of US streams, along with other hormone disruptors in pharmaceuticals.[90] These chemicals evade treatment plants and enter the water from home septic systems. Of the Boulder Creek Watershed in Colorado, the USGS writes, "Although it is difficult to assess the potential for adverse ecological effects of such complex chemical mixtures in the wastewater-affected part of Boulder Creek, native fish populations were found to exhibit endocrine disruption, including low male-to-female sex ratio and fish having both female and male reproductive organs (gonadal intersex)."[91]

Triclosan is unavoidable, and what's more—unnecessary. Studies have shown that regular soap and water is just as effective at preventing illness as triclosan-loaded soaps. Other countries have taken definitive steps in recent years to ban or greatly restrict the use of triclosan in products, to prevent any further accumulation and potential harm to human health and the natural world. In March 2010, the EU announced it would prohibit the use of triclosan in any products that came in contact with food; the EU had already moved to restrict the amount of triclosan in cosmetics. Canada, meanwhile, insisted in 2009 that manufacturers include warning labels on triclosan-containing cosmetics, stating that "the product is not to be used by children under the age of 12." Following consumer advisories regarding triclosan in Denmark, Norway, and Sweden in 2000, which warned that these products "can lead to adverse environmental and health effects," the use of triclosan in Denmark fell by 54 percent between 2000 and 2004.[92] Triclosan's own manufacturer, Ciba/BASF, recommended the restriction, saying that it "does not consider the use of the substance in plastics intended to come into contact with food to be appropriate any more."[93]

Compare this to the US, where the EPA has the authority to restrict triclosan in specific products like children's toys when manufacturer claims do not meet with the agency's approval, but a triclosan fact sheet released by Massachusetts Representative Ed Markey (D) found that "if the same manufacturer made the same toys but did not advertise the toys as being anti-bacterial, manufacturers wouldn't even have to disclose the triclosan the toys contain." The only way for the EPA to regulate exposure to triclosan, he concluded, "would be to prohibit its use in all plastics or in specific types of products, such as those intended for use by vulnerable populations (i.e., children) and in all plastics intended to come into contact with food."[94] In April 2010, Markey—the chairman of the Energy and Environment Subcommittee of the Energy and Commerce Committee—sent a letter to thirteen leading manufacturers of triclosan-containing products, including Proctor & Gamble, Rubbermaid, and Colgate-Palmolive, urging them to voluntarily stop using triclosan in their products.[95]

Absent labeling requirements or effective federal policies to limit chemical exposure from products, there is little protection for pregnant women, babies, and young children. Depending on manufacturers to voluntarily do the right thing is a national policy fraught with pitfalls. Even when the dangerous health and environmental impacts are known, restricting the use of chemicals in consumer products under the lax regulations of TSCA, or waiting until enough independent studies are funded that show conclusive harm, will keep real reform always out of reach. The only sane strategy is to undertake the kind of massive chemical reform seen in Europe—to set standards for all chemicals, existing or new, based on current health and environmental data, following a precautionary approach that considers, in every case, whether safer alternatives are available.

One researcher who spoke during the 2011 teleconference on autism and chemical exposures hosted by Safer Chemicals, Healthy Families was Dr. Lisa Huguenin, who holds a PhD in Environmental Science/Exposure Measurement and Assessment from Rutgers University and the University of Medicine and Dentistry of New Jersey, and specializes in environmental exposures. She also has a son with autism, and admitted that despite her training and knowledge of chemicals, she nonetheless felt "helpless" when her son began rapidly losing skills at the age of eighteen months. "Gone was his ability to hold a crayon and scribble," Dr. Huguenin says. "Gone was his amazing ability to kick a soccer ball and jump. Gone was his ability to say 'mommy' and 'daddy.' It was heart-wrenching." Following an autism diagnosis at age two, her son Harrison's health continued to rapidly deteriorate. "My son was experiencing severe gastrointestinal issues and was constantly sick," she continued. "He began to self-limit his diet and eventually stopped eating, falling rapidly off the growth charts." Not only did Harrison have autism, but he was also eventually diagnosed with severe food allergies, immune problems, and asthma. "To this day," she says, "he is unable to eat most food and gets nutrition from a formula provided by his doctor." All of her son's conditions, Dr. Huguenin noted, have been tied to environmental exposures, though of course she could not pinpoint in her particular case which exposures might have played a role. Anything and everything seemed suspect. "I worried about sulfates used to bathe my son, the shampoo I used for his cradle cap, the sealants that we put on his teeth," she says. "I worried about the fact that we recently resealed our deck, and that Harrison had chewed on his Thomas the Tank Engine toy that was eventually recalled for lead. I worried because my father and my husband's father both worked in the chemical industry and wondered if take-home exposures that my husband and I may have been exposed to when we were children were somehow involved. I worried that maybe our parents' exposures prior to our being born somehow affected us."[96]

Her experience with chemical exposures and their health consequences provided little comfort when it came to protecting her own family. Despite the fact that her family regularly tested their water and used environmentally friendly cleaners and paints without volatile organic compounds, she realized that when it came to environmental exposures, too much was out of her control. This was particularly true in regards to children's products like Thomas the Tank Engine toys from China, 1.5 million of which were recalled in 2007 because of high lead levels in the paint.[97] Toys like this make it to store shelves before undergoing safety testing only to be recalled later, after the health damage has been done. In the case of the much-beloved (and often high-priced) Thomas trains, lead was discovered in the paint beginning in 2005, nearly two and a half years before the manufacturer's voluntary recall.[98] And Dr. Huguenin described another disturbing safety slip-up regarding an arts and crafts toy she had purchased for her son, also made in China, called Aqua Dots—a toy involving hundreds of brightly colored beads that, if ingested, converted to gamma-hydroxy butyrate (GHB), a dangerous substance also used as a "date rape" drug. Two children swallowed Aqua Dots beads, vomited, and fell into a coma, prompting the 2007 recall of 4.2 million craft kits.[99] "This toy should have never been on the shelf—[but only] because the reaction to the ingestion of these beads was rather fast or acute this toy was able to be identified as a hazard and pulled from the shelf," Dr. Hugeunin says. But, she asks: "How about the toys and products that may have chemicals in them that . . . have more long-term effects, such as carcinogens, neurotoxins, or endocrine disruptors? Effects that we may not see for years or possibly generations? With TSCA in its current form," she says, "I still have questions and worry about the safety of the products I buy and I use every day. . . . TSCA reform is needed. There is no plausible reason for any chemical that goes into a product, especially a children's item, not to be thoroughly tested prior to its use."[100]

SEVEN

Unanswered Questions
Avoiding Toxins and Taking Action

The known danger of inadequately tested chemicals, chemical compounds, and heavy metals to children's health and development is enough to leave any parent with grave worries. Sharon will always carry concerns about her possible exposure to lead paint and other pollutants common to urban environments during her pregnancy with James. She'll always wonder how the power plant and highway emissions, abandoned factories, and warehouses leaking industrial solvents may have interacted with her son's genetic predisposition, her undeniable family history of the disorder, perhaps prompting his pre-term birth, his developmental delays, and his autism. Though the investigation into contaminants in her community's water supply was inconclusive, Bobbie will always worry that disinfectant byproducts or trihalomethanes she inhaled from the water in her home triggered autism in her youngest daughter and son. Then again, because the investigating agencies did not actually test her household dust, her floors, her tap water,

147

or take blood or urine samples from her family, she has many questions that will never be answered about which chemical exposures could have played a role. And in Wisconsin, Cindy will always remain concerned about the lead- and mercury-spewing coal plant a couple miles up the road. She'll never know for certain where that contamination fits into her larger family story—a family whose male members exhibit signs of Asperger's. She'll keep combing through her youngest son's medical history and her detailed journal of his development, searching for clues that pinpoint when and how he changed from a responsive child into a withdrawn, obsessive, tantrum-prone child with autism. Was it her age at the time of his birth? The drugs administered during pregnancy?

The increased studies of how chemicals, heavy metals, and drugs and synthetic hormones administered during pregnancy and childbirth may be contributing to rising rates of autism have left us, thus far, with only clues. But they are compelling nonetheless. The growing number of children with autism, a condition that requires, in many cases, a lifetime of care and medical expense, is not simply the result of a genetic aberration that we are helpless to prevent. Rather, it is evidence of where we as a society have gone wrong in protecting children's health, where we have overstepped the bounds of safety and allowed dangerous chemicals to spread throughout the natural world and build up in our tissues, bloodstreams, and breast milk without consideration of their long-term consequences.

We know definitively that there are a greater number of chemicals in our bodies than ever before, and that developing infants are exposed to these chemicals in greater numbers than their parents. In the past, we may have assumed that the chemicals in our products served a purpose—in the case of BPA, to keep our canned food from perishing; in the case of phthalates in plastic, to give our food storage integrity; in the case of PBDEs, to keep our furniture and electronics from being prone to catch fire; in the case of formaldehyde, to keep our wood decks, siding, and furniture from being damaged by moisture. Now we know that these protections are minor compared to the danger such exposures represent to vulnerable babies.

The story of an average US family is one of the best illustrations of just how far our chemical hubris has led us. In 2005 the *Oakland Tribune* conducted an investigation in which a California couple from the Bay Area, Michele Hammond and her husband, Jeremiah Holland, consented to have their blood, urine, and hair, along with samples from their two children, Mikaela and Rowan, tested for chemical concentrations. It was the first study to measure the levels of flame retardants in a family. In addition to PBDEs, researchers analyzed their samples for the presence of metals, PCBs, phthalates, and perfluorinated acid used in Teflon and other nonstick products. They found everything but arsenic, with the children's concentrations often registering higher than that of their parents. This was particularly true in the case of flame retardants. Researchers found that Michele and Jeremiah had about 100 ppb of PBDEs in their bloodstreams; Mikaela had 500 ppb, and Rowan had close to 700 ppb. The researchers suspect that the children's greater exposure was a result of their ingesting the chemical by inhaling household dust.[1] A Canadian study found that children are likely to ingest one hundred times the PBDEs that their parents do, and our national failure to restrict these chemicals means they are present in our children's bodies at increasingly alarming rates. In 2008 the ATSDR wrote that, "levels of lower brominated PBDEs in the general population of the United States continue to rise. The US levels are 10-100 times higher than levels in individuals living in Europe."[2] Because flame retardants take up residence in the body's fat, breast milk is a major chemical conduit from mother to child. *The Oakland Tribune* reported that using known estimates for PBDE concentrations in breast milk, Rowan, who was still breastfeeding at age two and a half, was likely getting "130 ppb from his mother every day." Naturally, his mother was angry. She now questions the fact that her son has always been small for his age and is prone to acting out. She questions how her commitment to breastfeeding might have unwittingly harmed her son. "It's sad I have to even ponder that I might be damaging my child by breastfeeding," Michele told the paper. "Why do I have to feel there's anything negative about breast milk?"[3]

We've come a long way in our understanding of autism since the misguided 1950s theory of the "refrigerator mother" was put to rest. But now, in the twenty-first century, we are again in the position of questioning mothers. Engaged, caring moms who breastfeed their infants might be harming their children in the course of providing milk that's tainted with harmful chemicals. Even the most conscientious moms, those who buy only certified organic products and food items, and use homemade, nontoxic cleaners, will still pass the chemicals that have accumulated in their bodies to their infants during the course of breastfeeding. Leading neuroscientist Dr. Merzenich wonders whether mothers living in areas of high toxic contamination will begin having their milk tested for pollutants before determining if it is safe to breastfeed their infants. "When we delivered PCBs to the mother, the mother delivered it to the infant by nursing," he says. "What a thing that a mother could be poisoning her infant by nursing her. What a crazy world we live in."[4]

Our world is chemically contaminated, the health of our children compromised, and there is little information and inadequate regulation to keep us safe. It is unacceptable that the ATSDR, in its fact sheet on flame retardants, for example, states that "Nothing definite is known about the health effects of PBDEs in people," but admits later in the same paragraph that "Preliminary findings from short-term animal studies suggest that some PBDEs might impair the immune system." The agency openly admits that some PBDEs cause cancer in animals, but that the "lower brominated PBDEs," to which humans are most often exposed, "have not yet been tested for cancer."[5] The connection between chemical exposures and rising autism, allergy and asthma rates, early puberty, child-onset diabetes and obesity, and attention deficit and other behavioral disorders has been ignored for far too long. Overhauling our national chemical policy is imperative, and politicians must be pressured to challenge the chemical industry.

The necessary impetus may come from an ambitious new study called the National Children's Study that is currently taking place in more than one hundred locations in nearly every state in the union. The study will look at a broad range of environmental influences— including air, water, sound, family dynamics, community, and cultural influences—to discover how these factors, acting separately and together, impact the health and wellbeing of children, from before birth to age twenty-one.

Though it was established in 2000 as part of the Children's Health Act, the National Children's Study was still in the recruitment stage by 2010, with researchers trying to find families willing to undergo scrutiny of their habits and the health of their children over multiple decades. Initially, this recruitment effort began in medical clinics, with health care providers encouraging pregnant women to participate. But that strategy carries its own inherent bias, says Dr. Patricia O'Campo, a social epidemiologist at the Centre for Research on Inner City Health at the University of Toronto, St. Michael's Hospital, and a federal advisory committee member for the study. "Often, if you go to a particular clinic, the population there is not representative of the surrounding area," Dr. O'Campo says. "Some clinics primarily take Medicaid or private patients." Trained recruiters have had to go door to door in search of willing families, as well as sending letters, calling people at home, and directing people to the study's website to win them over. The response rate has been much slower than anticipated. "Despite finding eligible women," Dr. O'Campo says, "not all are saying 'yes.'"[6] *The New York Times* profiled a mother from Queens, New York, named Alejandra (her last name withheld for confidentiality reasons) who only warily agreed to participate after repeated requests from the government scientists who visited. Agreeing meant that she would allow researchers to collect vaginal fluid, toenail clippings, breast milk, her placenta, and her baby's first feces, among many other samples. It also meant that Alejandra would have to answer questions across twenty-one years related to everything from her mental health to her use of alcohol and drugs.[7] But assuming that the sought-after number of pregnant women agreeing to these terms can be reached, the National Children's Study will accomplish what other smaller studies connecting chemicals to children's health have not. Any evidence of harm discovered will no longer be deemed "inconclusive" or impossible to extrapolate because of small sampling size. If the study looks at the environmental impacts and outcomes of one hundred thousand infants across the US, it will have, as the study's website says, "a statistically valid population that will permit both generalizations about the nation as a whole and detailed analysis of specific communities and subpopulations."[8]

In May 2010, the Mount Sinai Medical Center in New York launched its own specialized study of the connection between environmental chemicals and autism and other learning disabilities called the Autism and Learning Disabilities Discovery and Prevention Project. Their first goal is to rank the 1,200 industrial chemicals that are known to be toxic to the adult brain and in lab animals, but that have yet to be tested for impact on developing human brains. They will zero in on the chemicals most widely distributed in the homes and environments of children and pregnant women, and those that turn up most often in blood samples as found in national surveys done by the CDC. Maternal blood samples, cord blood, and placental tissue samples collected at delivery will provide clues as to what exposures, genetic susceptibilities, and epigenetic markers have contributed to autism and other learning disabilities.[9] The study's findings will be instrumental in supporting the more comprehensive efforts of the National Children's Study.

With the substantial, verifiable, cross-tested data from the National Children's Study and the Autism and Learning Disabilities Discovery and Prevention Project in hand, the EPA will finally have the legislative authority to ban dangerous chemicals from manufacture and sale. It's not a perfect process, and the time for these definitive answers still lies far into the coming decades. While it may be of little comfort to parents planning families in the present day, the impetus to finally connect the dots between industrial chemicals and autism and other children's health disorders and diseases marks a major step forward in shifting the focus of autism research from genetics to environmental causes.

In the meantime, parents can take preventative action to limit chemical exposures, particularly during pregnancy and throughout their children's early years. Pregnant and nursing women, would-be moms, and young children may choose to avoid eating fish with high mercury content, particularly "big fish" like shark, swordfish, king mackerel, and tilefish. Albacore or "white" tuna also has more mercury than light tuna, the EPA notes, so the agency recommends no more than six ounces of albacore tuna a week during pregnancy (about one meal's worth) and no more than twelve ounces for light tuna. Beyond that, anyone planning to eat fish they've caught themselves may check with local advisories first. If no advisories have been issued, the EPA says that pregnant and nursing women, would-be mothers, and young children may eat up to six ounces (one meal) of self-caught fish in a week, adding, "but don't consume any other fish during that week."[10]

Parents may also—as many have already begun to do—switch to organic fruits and vegetables, or if this is not feasible, thoroughly wash and peel any nonorganic produce to limit pesticides coming from diet. Not all fruits and vegetables are equal when it comes to pesticide residues. The EWG produces a yearly updated "Shopper's Guide to Pesticides in Produce," in which fifty-three fruits and vegetables are ranked from most contaminated (apples) to least contaminated (onions), so cost-conscious parents can choose which items are most important to buy organic. The rankings are based on pesticide residue data from the US Department of Agriculture (USDA) and the FDA, and reveal that many fresh, presumably healthy foods are tainted with a variety of pesticides, even after being washed or peeled. The EWG website notes, "Because all produce has been thoroughly cleaned before analysis, washing a fruit or vegetable would not change its rank in the EWG's Shopper's Guide . . . [but] if you don't wash conventional produce, the risk of ingesting pesticides is even greater than reflected by USDA test data."[11] In terms of chemical combinations present on a single piece of fruit, studies found that conventional peaches contain combinations of fifty-seven different chemicals, the most of any produce; apples had fifty-six chemicals, and raspberries had fifty-one. According to the EWG, celery, spinach, sweet bell peppers, potatoes, lettuce, and greens (kale and collards) are the vegetables most likely to retain pesticide contamination. In addition to onions, the list of "clean" fruits and vegetables includes sweet corn, pineapples, avocado, asparagus, sweet peas, mangoes, eggplant, domestic cantaloupe, kiwi, cabbage, watermelon, sweet potatoes, grapefruit, and mushrooms.[12] For quick reference, the "Dirty Dozen" fruits and vegetables with the most pesticides that should be purchased organic and the "Clean 15" fruits and vegetables with the least pesticide residues are available as a printable PDF from the EWG website or as a free app for the iPhone, iPod Touch, or iPad.

How food is prepared matters too, as chemicals can easily be introduced into meals by cooking food in Teflon-coated pots and pans or heating it in plastic containers or Teflon-coated packaging in the microwave or oven. Teflon and other nonstick coatings contain perfluorooctanoic acid which, the EPA writes, "is found at very low levels both in the environment and in the blood of the general US population, and causes developmental and other adverse effects in laboratory animals." In fact, the agency's science advisory board called PFOA a "likely human carcinogen," since it has been linked to cancers of the breast, testes, pancreas, and liver in animal studies.[13] What's more, a 2007 study found that infants with higher levels of PFOA and the related chemical perfluorooctane sulfonate (PFO) had lower birth weights and smaller head circumferences. The chemical compounds were so ubiquitous that PFOA was detected in the bloodstreams in 100 percent of infants researchers studied, and PFO in 99 percent.[14] Even the weak protections offered by TSCA bowed under the increasing evidence that the chemical was much more harmful than had been previously disclosed, and in 2004, the EPA took administrative action against DuPont, the chemical manufacturer that produces Teflon. The company's manufacturing processes had allowed PFOA to contaminate drinking water, accumulate in the environment, and take up residence in the bloodstreams of most Americans. In 2005, DuPont was forced to pay $10.25 million for violating federal environmental statutes, the largest civil penalty the agency has ever received.[15] But while the EPA has initiated efforts to reduce emissions of PFOA and to develop safer alternatives, it has not issued any restrictions on the use of Teflon, which contains trace amounts of PFOA, for cooking or consumer use. The chemical is also present in Gore-Tex clothing, carpets, couches, and many other stain-, grease-, and water-resistant materials. It is also in the coated linings of some of Americans' favorite—but least healthy—foods, including microwave popcorn bags, frozen pizza packaging, and french fry containers.[16]

Consumers may cut back on PFOA exposure by popping corn with an air popper, cutting back on fast food runs, and avoiding packaged-for-heating foods in general, since companies are not required to disclose PFOA content on their labels. For cookware, the advocacy group Safer Chemicals, Healthy Families recommends using stainless steel, cast iron, or enameled pots and pans instead of Teflon. And to help consumers better understand the difficult-to-pronounce additives found on the ingredient labels of so many packaged foods, like acesulfame-k (an artificial sweetener that's two hundred times sweeter than sugar and found in diet sodas and baked goods) or butylated hydroxyanisole (an antioxidant that retards toxicity and is found in cereals, potato chips, and gum), the Center for Science in the Public Interest

(CSPI) offers a downloadable app for $0.99 called Chemical Cuisine that describes the history and potential health risks of more than 130 food additives. A green check mark indicates if an additive is safe, a red "x" indicates if it should be avoided. The complete details are also available on CSPI's website (and, for the record, both the above additives are on the to-be-avoided list).[17]

Where possible, plastic products, particularly those used for food storage and as beverage containers, should be kept to a minimum. Families should avoid washing plastic dishes and sippy cups in the dishwasher or using them to microwave food since chemicals like BPA can leach and contaminate food. Families should be particularly wary of transferring heated liquids like infant formula into BPA-containing bottles, or using plastic dishes that have become scratched or worn. A switch to stainless steel water bottles and glass and stainless steel storage containers is recommended. The US Department of Health and Human Services gives special note to canned, liquid infant formulas, many of which have been found to contain BPA. To limit an increase in BPA exposure, parents are advised not to heat these cans on the stove or in boiling water, but instead to run warm water over the outside of a bottle after the formula has been added (powdered formulas have not been found to contain similar levels of BPA).[18] With the voluntary elimination of BPA by major US bottle manufacturers, more than 90 percent of infant bottles for sale will not contain the chemical; of course, parents should still be sure to check labels and to replace older plastic bottles.

Safer Chemicals, Healthy Families has developed its own set of steps to help families reduce their BPA levels by 60 percent or more in just three days, based on studies of five families, the results of which were published in *Environmental Health Perspectives*. A total of twenty family members took part in a "dietary intervention," in which participants ate their usual diets, followed by three days of eating "fresh foods that were not canned or packaged in plastic," and then returned to their usual diets again. Researchers took urine samples throughout and analyzed them for changes in BPA and DEHP concentrations. The differences were dramatic: Following the dietary intervention, average concentrations of BPA dropped by 66 percent and DEHP metabolites by 53 to56 percent, the study found.[19]

Because the greatest exposures were coming from food packaging, the advice centers on changes to diet. Families are advised to switch to fresh fruits and vegetables where possible, and frozen foods, as opposed to canned, where it's not. Instead of buying canned beans, the group suggests soaking dried beans, and freezing extra to have a ready supply. Canned foods that are acidic, salty, or fatty are to be particularly avoided, as these have been found to contain the highest levels of BPA leaching from can linings. A Safer Chemicals, Healthy Families downloadable wallet card includes the following canned foods to avoid: coconut milk, soup, meat, vegetables, meals (like ravioli), juice, fish, beans, meal-replacement drinks, and fruit.[20] Eating out less often is also important, particularly at restaurants that don't serve fresh foods. Finally, the group encourages families to consider a French-press coffee pot, as "home coffee makers may have polycarbonate-based water tanks and phthalate-based tubing." Phthalates in plastic—which were once found in everything from teethers to rattles to plastic toys and bottle nipples—have been outlawed in infant and children's products in the US. But the law just took effect in February of 2009, so to avoid exposure, parents should start fresh with plastic products for newborns, and avoid used baby products that may have been sold before the ban took effect, including plastic cribs or plastic-covered crib mattresses. The baby's room as a whole should be approached with a chemical-free mindset—using low- or no-VOC paint on the walls; buying furniture that does not contain formaldehyde (when in doubt, avoid particle board altogether); and limiting electronic equipment, such as computers, stereos, and televisions, in the baby's room. As Dr. Merzenich explains, electronic equipment—particularly older models—often contains brominated flame retardants like PBDEs that can be released into household dust and later inhaled. And while phthalates may be less likely to turn up in new plastic toys and teethers, they are still found in baby shampoo, powder, and lotion, often hidden inside fragrance ingredients, which are not disclosed on labels. Many of these products are largely unnecessary for infants, who require only the mildest washing, but they can also be replaced with products clearly labeled "phthalate-free" or those made without fragrances and with certified organic ingredients. Natural oils (as opposed to petroleum-based mineral oils), including Vitamin E, safflower oil, and olive oil, are a safe replacement for lotions, and often provide better relief for a baby's dry, sensitive skin.

Natural replacements are also recommended for adults' personal care products and cosmetics. Often, in reaching for the products we are most familiar with—Dial soap, Revlon nail polish, Cover Girl lipstick—we don't stop to consider how the ingredients, which are often not disclosed, may be cause for concern. There is triclosan in antibacterial soaps; what the Campaign for Safe Cosmetics calls the "toxic trio," dibutyl phthalate, toluene, and formaldehyde, in nail polish; and lead in lipstick. The last issue is a major concern to lipstick lovers, particularly since anything on the lips can be easily and inadvertently ingested. But the Campaign for Safe Cosmetics tested thirty-three popular lipstick brands for lead content in 2007, and found that 61 percent of the samples contained lead, including those by L'Oreal, Cover Girl, and, even "a $24 tube of Dior Addict."After two years of the Campaign for Safe Cosmetics, consumers, and certain senators pressuring the FDA to investigate, the FDA finally conducted its own tests, and the results were even more alarming. Lead was found "in all of the lipsticks tested, ranging from 0.09 ppm [parts per million] to 3.06 ppm with an average value of 1.07 ppm."[21] Even lipsticks from presumed-to-be-natural brands like Body Shop and Burt's Bees contained lead. But the FDA, which admits it "has not set limits for contaminants, including lead, in cosmetics," concluded that lead in lipstick does not pose a health risk since lipstick is a "product intended for topical use," that "is only ingested incidentally and in very small quantities."[22] With the known neurological damage to a developing fetus that can come from lead exposure, even in small amounts, scientists have reached a very different conclusion: "No level of lead exposure appears to be 'safe' and even the current 'low' levels of exposure in children are associated with neurodevelopmental deficits [including reduced intelligence, poor academic performance, ADHD and antisocial behavior]," writes Dr. David Bellinger, a professor of environmental health at Harvard School of Public Health, in *Pediatrics*. The only safe course of action, he argues, is to prevent exposure.[23] A bill to ban lead in lipstick in California passed the state senate but died in the Assembly Health Committee in 2008 after intense lobbying pressure from the beauty industry, including representatives for Revlon, L'Oreal, and Johnson & Johnson.[24]

Since labels can't be trusted and laws offer little protection, the best hope for consumers looking to buy cosmetics and personal care products free of toxic chemicals and contaminants is to consult the EWG's Skin Deep Cosmetics Database, an online directory of more than sixty-five thousand products including suntan lotion, body lotion, soap, shampoo, toothpaste, nail polish, perfume, shaving cream, hair dye, and more. The organization has taken online ingredient lists from manufacturers, where available, and used them to rate products in terms of their potential health impacts. Each product has a "hazard" rating on a scale from one to ten, with ten being the most hazardous. Hazards taken into account include carcinogens, reproductive and developmental toxins, allergens, and immunotoxicity and use restrictions. The products have a separate "data availability rating" (no data, limited data, fair data, and so on) that "reflects how much scientists know—or don't know—about an ingredient's safety." Consumers may search for specific products by brand name, or they may scroll by product type to view products listed from least to most hazardous. Among baby shampoos, the highest hazard rating given was a "6" for Baby Magic Hair and Body Wash by Playtex Products, Inc., the ingredients of which registered high concerns for developmental and reproductive toxicity. Several lipstick brands were rated "tens," including Avon Pro-to-Go lipstick, Smashbox Lips Tinted Treatment, and Paula Dorf Lip Color For Lips.[25]

There are strategies for avoiding contamination from local water supplies, too. Women may reduce exposure to THMs and other toxins by allowing drinking water to remain in an uncovered pitcher in the refrigerator for several hours before drinking it; many of the THMs are volatile, and will evaporate. When taking showers, pregnant women may opt for cooler (as opposed to steamy) water temperatures, which will reduce inhalation and skin absorption. Opening a window or using a fan during showers can also help, and taking a bath as opposed to a shower reduces exposure even further. Keep in mind, too, that THM concentrations tend to be highest during the summer and early fall, when the right condition for chlorine to interact with organic matter in the water, giving rise to THMs, is at its peak.[26]

Many communities across the country have contaminated drinking water as a result of local pollution and out-of-date plumbing. Lead has been found in the water of New York City homes built prior to 1961 with lead service lines, as well as homes built prior to 1987 with plumbing connected by lead solder. Tests by officials in New York in 2010 found that 14 percent of tap water samples exceeded allowable lead levels.[27] Lead levels in the water are highest first thing in the morning, or after returning home from school or work, when water had been sitting in the pipes for hours. For that reason, the city's Department of Environmental Protection issued a "Run Your Tap" campaign, advising homeowners to "Run your tap for at least 30 seconds, until the water is noticeably colder, before using it for drinking, cooking or making baby formula any time the water in the faucet has stood for several hours."

And the department advised using only cold water for drinking or cooking since hot water takes up lead more readily.[28]

When the Natural Resources Defense Council (NRDC) studied water supplies across nineteen diverse US cities in 2003, they found a host of other concerning contaminants in addition to lead and THMs. Some drinking supplies were home to pathogens like chloriform bacteria, which can be particularly harmful to children and those with compromised immune systems; arsenic; the pesticide atrazine (present in the drinking water of one million Americans); and perchlorate from rocket fuel (found in the water supplies of more than twenty million Americans). Cities with the poorest drinking water quality from the NRDC's "What's on Tap?" report included Albuquerque, New Mexico; Boston, Massachusetts; Phoenix, Arizona; and Fresno and San Francisco, California.[29] The first step for concerned families is to have their home water tested so they know precisely what contaminants they need to treat. Armed with that information, homeowners can reduce a good number of water-based contaminants with a home filtering system, particularly a carbon or charcoal filter combined with a reverse osmosis system that moves the water through a membrane from a more concentrated to a more dilute solution. The National Sanitation Foundation (NSF) walks consumers through a range of options for treating home water systems, from point-of-entry systems installed after the water meter that filter all a home's water, to point-of-use systems that can be plumbed in or mounted to an existing or auxiliary faucet. Pitchers for filtering water work, too, though are obviously more limited in terms of how much water they can hold. The NSF website has a database for certified water filtration products to make comparison shopping easier.

Perhaps one of the easiest ways for homeowners to rid their home environments of potentially dangerous chemicals is to revamp their cleaning habits. Ingredient disclosure—and not claims of "green" or "biodegradable" on the front of cleaners—is key to choosing safer products. The companies that fully disclose their ingredients, such as Seventh Generation and Ecover, are not hiding dangerous chemical additives like toxic butyl cellosolve, a hidden ingredient in the Simple Green line of cleaners that causes red blood cell destruction and minor birth defects in lab animals.[30] Shoppers should look for plant-based and oil-based cleaners, and should avoid disinfectants that introduce dangerous pesticides into the home, according to Carole LeBlanc, lab director of the Toxic Use Reduction Institute at University of Massachusetts, Lowell. LeBlanc adds that the term "nontoxic," which is unregulated, is meaningless. The safest—and cheapest—way for families to clean up their cleaning habits is to replace store-bought cleaners with homemade versions. A mixture of distilled white vinegar and water in a spray bottle is an effective glass cleaner and spray for cleaning kitchen spills and household sinks, and distilled white vinegar can be mixed with baking soda for a homemade scouring cleanser to remove stains surrounding drains and stubborn grease stains. Even the youngest family members can help scrub and wash without worry when you make your own cleaners.

Pregnant women are also advised to avoid handling insect sprays and flea and tick solutions, or to switch to less harmful products like boric acid or an even safer solution of white vinegar and water to spray on pets. A light application of diatomaceous earth (made from the fossils of freshwater organisms) may be used on floors and rugs after thorough vacuuming. When any pesticide treatment is performed in the home, the University of Washington recommends that all food containers, utensils, and toys be removed from the vicinity, and everything should be washed before children and pets return.[31]

These piecemeal measures provide a few avenues of parental control to at least limit any additional chemicals being brought into the home. Of course, chemical contamination is so widespread both in the environment and in our bodies that complete avoidance is impossible. In addition to undertaking preventive measures at home, the best we can do for our children's health is to join national efforts to pass meaningful chemical reform. The nonprofit Healthy Child, Healthy World is leading these efforts. Its website connects visitors with legislative efforts for chemical reform and provides information about the dangers of chemical exposures, as does the website for EWG, which includes information on how to e-mail representatives on key health and toxin issues and provides exhaustive data on the chemical makeup of cosmetics, drinking water, and sunscreens. The Natural Resources Defense Council is particularly invested in the fight for cleaner water, both for people and wildlife. The council is pushing for better water monitoring and a phase-out of atrazine, a harmful pesticide that causes hormone disruption and immune system impairment in animals, and which was found "in 80 percent of drinking water samples taken in 153 public water systems" in 2010 testing. The group has also alerted the public and legislators to the ways that chemical companies have sought to undermine the protections of the Clean Water Act, which they call "The EPA's only tool to protect water quality and fish, wildlife and human health from pesticide contamination."[32] The Natural Resources Defense Council's March 2011 report notes that chemical companies are pushing for allowances under the EPA's Federal Insecticide, Fungicide, and Rodenticide Act (FIFRA) exclusively, the labeling requirements of which are not sufficient to protect waterways from pesticide contamination.[33] Like many nonprofits working at the intersection of environmental exposure and human health, the group Safer Chemicals, Healthy Families has made reforming TSCA its primary mission. The group provides legislative updates on the history and progress of the Safer Chemicals Act and an easy way to contact your representatives for support. They were instrumental, along with the Campaign for Safe Cosmetics, in getting the Safe Cosmetics Act introduced in Congress in June 2011, to ensure that personal care and cosmetic products are free of "lead, reproductive toxins, and cancer-causing chemicals like formaldehyde."[34] The current legislation guiding the FDA's governing of cosmetics—which the Safe Cosmetics Act would replace—has not been updated in more than seventy years. The Safer Chemicals, Healthy Families and Campaign for Safe Cosmetics websites connect visitors with multiple ways to contact legislators and ask them to co-sponsor the proposed law.

With the help of these and other advocacy groups, it is possible to move from feeling helpless to empowered. Families may track which bills pertaining to children's health and chemical regulation are in the works, sign a petition, or e-mail a senator or representative with a few simple clicks. Making chemical regulation a national priority requires an informed—and outraged—citizenry. The environmental clues in the autism mystery are in the process of being discovered, but we can't afford to wait for final conclusions as our collective body burden of chemicals climbs along with the rising rates of autism and other diseases and disorders. Only by banning and restricting unproven or known-to-be-dangerous chemicals will we begin to see these chemical concentrations—from BPA to flame retardants—in our blood and breast milk fall, as has happened in Europe, Canada, and Japan.

Thanks to states' moving to restrict chemicals of concern in the marketplace, stores are opting to remove worrisome items from store shelves. And the public's growing skepticism of products from cleaners to cosmetics to cookware has left the chemical industry at a crossroads with nothing to gain, financially or perception-wise, from clinging to secrets. Andy Igrejas, the national campaign director for Safer Chemicals, Healthy Families, has watched the fight over increased chemical regulation play out in the halls of Congress and says the industry as a whole will benefit from embracing comprehensive chemical reform. "It's a fundamental choice for industry," Igrejas says. "They've gotten so addicted to their K Street power, which is so effective at blocking things and grinding things to a halt—it's almost worked too well. Now they're really faced with the idea that they're not credible with the public and that's having an effect in the marketplace . . . they could face a system where states are regulating them, Europe's regulating them, and all they've done is prevented a strong federal role from restoring credibility to the marketplace."[35]

In a world of protected industry secrets, outdated materials, and toxic landfills, parents do not have the ability to know exactly what is in the products their families use, the buildings their children frequent, or the canned food they eat. That responsibility belongs with manufacturers, who must begin proving that their products are safe, not only for adults, but for pregnant women and the developing children inside their wombs whose brains are just beginning to make the neural connections that will impact how they function, learn, trust, and love. It is immoral to allow questionable chemicals to be manufactured and used. That certain exposures, whether combined with each other or in combination with genetic susceptibilities, are implicated in rising autism rates should be all the information we need to insist on new legislation that provides protection, finally, for those who can't speak for themselves.

RESOURCES

❖

Organizations Involved in Autism and/or Toxin Research, Advocacy, and Education

Autism Society
4340 East-West Highway, Suite 350
Bethesda, MD 20814
(800) 328-8476
www.autism-society.org

"The nation's leading grassroots autism organization," the Autism Society is a resource both for understanding autism and following the latest research, including research connecting autism to environmental toxins.

Autism Speaks
1 East 33rd Street, 4th Floor
New York, NY 10016
(212) 252-8584
www.autismspeaks.org
contactus@autismspeaks.org

Autism Speaks is an autism science and advocacy organization that supports research into "the causes, prevention, treatments and a cure for autism" and provides information and support for individuals with autism and families seeking answers. Autism Speaks provides resources specifically geared toward adults with autism, information about work opportunities as well as "Family Support Tool Kits" for parents, siblings, grandparents and friends.

Campaign for Safe Cosmetics
www.safecosmetics.org
info@safecosmetics.org

A coalition between health and environmental nonprofits that's working to secure "the corporate, regulatory, and legislative reforms necessary to eliminate dangerous chemicals from cosmetics and personal care products." Follow bills in progress, watch informative videos, and find out which brands you can trust.

Center for Health, Environment & Justice
www.chej.org

Founded by activist Lois Gibbs after the toxic disaster at Love Canal, CHEJ has helped craft national policies related to protecting community health, from the Superfund Program to Right-to-Know laws regarding toxic exposures. They've helped major corporations like McDonald's move away from harmful packaging like Styrofoam and convinced Microsoft to turn from PVC plastic. One recent initiative was "Childproofing Our Communities."

Center for Science in the Public Interest
1220 L St. NW, Suite 300
Washington, DC 20005
(202) 332-9110
www.cspinet.org

The CSPI advocates for "nutrition and health, food safety, alcohol policy, and sound science." They are working to improve food safety laws and encourage eco-friendly diets, and their Chemical Cuisine online guide (and downloadable app) is an invaluable resource for learning the health impacts of all those chemicals and additives on food labels.

Children's Environmental Health Network
110 Maryland Ave. NE Suite 402
Washington, DC 20002
(202) 543-4033
www.cehn.org
cehn@cehn.org

An organization working to "protect the developing child from environmental health hazard and promote a healthier environment." They track children's health news related to toxic exposures, host events, and provide information on healthy homes.

The Collaborative on Health and the Environment
c/o Commonweal
PO Box 316
Bolinas, CA 94924
www.healthandenvironment.org
info@healthandenvironment.org

An "international partnership committed to strengthening the scientific and public dialogue on the impact of environmental factors on human health and catalyzing initiatives to address these concerns." The CHE website features a comprehensive Toxicant and Disease Database, which can be searched by disease or toxin, and launched an autism working group, CHE Autism, in 2009.

Columbia Center for Children's Environmental Health
722 W. 168th St., 12th Floor
New York, NY 10032
(212) 304 7180
ccceh.hs.columbia.edu
cccehcolumbia@gmail.com

Run by the Columbia University Mailman School of Public Health, CCCEH provides expert information and research about environmental hazards like pesticides, phthalates, and mercury and related health risks. A special tab for parents and families offers ways to reduce exposures and "green" your home life.

Environment & Human Health, Inc.
1191 Ridge Rd.
North Haven, CT 06473
(203) 248-6582
www.ehhi.org
info@ehhi.org

A nonprofit "dedicated to protecting human health from environmental harms through research, education and the promotion of sound public policy."

Environmental Defense Fund
257 Park Ave. South
New York, NY 10010
(800) 684-3322
www.edf.org

EDF is "dedicated to protecting the environmental rights of all people, including future generations. Among these rights are access to clean air and water, healthy and nourishing food, and flourishing ecosystems." The group actively seeks to bring about chemical reform, and their "I Am Not a Guinea Pig" campaign (www.notaguineapig.org) gives people easy-to-access information about toxins of concern, fixing the law, and research updates.

Environmental Health News
www.environmentalhealthnews.org

Published by Environmental Health Sciences, it's a foundation-funded journalism organization and a one-stop site for the latest news reports and research releases related to health and toxins.

Environmental Working Group
1436 U St. NW, Suite 100
Washington, DC 20009
(202) 667-6982
www.ewg.org

One of the most passionate voices for protecting people's health, Environmental Working Group provides the data and studies that show us the harm of everyday toxic exposures and the degree to which our bodies (and those of our newborns and children) are polluted. They offer a comprehensive chemical index, a guide to pesticides in produce, the Skin Deep cosmetic safety database, a sunscreen safety guide, health tips on everything from personal care products to preventing cancer, and regular legislative and research updates.

Friends of the Earth
1100 15th St. NW, 11th Floor
Washington, DC 20005
(202) 783-7400 or toll-free (877) 843-8687
www.foe.org

Friends of the Earth describe themselves as "progressive environmental advocates who pull no punches and speak sometimes uncomfortable truths to power." They challenge dirty fossil fuels, nanotechnology, and dangerous chemicals from flame retardants to endocrine disruptors. Their Safe Kids Campaign focuses specifically on advancing legislation that would remove dangerous chemicals from products kids are exposed to.

Natural Resources Defense Council
40 W. 20th St.
New York, NY 10011
(212) 727-2700
www.nrdc.org

NRDC is one of the largest grassroots environmental organizations that works both to protect wildlife and people. They are particularly effective at advocating for cleaner water and to curb pollution, and their online "Smarter Living" tab offers a wealth of information for anyone looking for healthy alternatives whether in food, sunscreens, kitchenware, or pet care.

Our Stolen Future
www.ourstolenfuture.org

A website that arose out of a book by the same name, Our Stolen Future tracks the latest research and policies regarding endocrine disruptors like BPA.

Pesticide Action Network
49 Powell St., Suite 500
San Francisco, CA 94102
(415) 981-1771
www.panna.org

PAN North America "works to replace the use of hazardous pesticides with ecologically sound and socially just alternatives." They are vocal advocates for safer school buildings and playgrounds, track the latest research related to children's health and toxins, and act as a media watchdog.

Physicians for Social Responsibility
1875 Connecticut Ave. NW, Suite 1012
Washington, DC 20009
(202) 667-4260
www.psr.org

PSR is "the medical and public health voice working to prevent the use or spread of nuclear weapons and to slow, stop and reverse global warming and the toxic degradation of the environment." They offer a Pediatric Environmental Health Toolkit for health professionals and provide research tools for parents interested in environmental health topics.

Safer Chemicals, Healthy Families
www.saferchemicals.org

SCHF is dedicated to passing meaningful chemical reform at the federal level, enlisting the support of such A-listers as Jessica Alba to draw attention to their cause. They also provide great tips for families on reducing toxic exposures, ridding one's diet of BPA, and protecting one's reproductive health. Their "Meet the Chemicals" series featuring cartoon characters like BPA and Flame Retardants, along with a helpful video, breaks down which toxins to avoid, and why.

Women's Voices for the Earth
114 W. Pine St., PO Box 8743
Missoula, MT 59807
(406) 543-3747
www.womensvoices.org
womensvoices@womensvoices.org

A "national organization that works to eliminate toxic chemicals that impact women's health by changing consumer behaviors, corporate practices and government policies." Initiatives include safe cleaning products, safe cosmetics and chemicals to avoid.

ACKNOWLEDGMENTS

❖

I am grateful for the love and support of my family and in-laws who provided the space and encouragement that made writing this book possible, and especially for my mother, Mary, who first taught me to cherish words. I am particularly grateful to my husband, Jerry, and daughter, Eleanore, who have given me countless reasons to smile and persevere despite working through so many pre-dawn mornings. And I am inspired by my work family at E – *The Environmental Magazine*, a publication that has taught me both the importance of environmental issues and the great things that can be accomplished by a small group of dedicated individuals.

To the parents who opened their doors and hearts to me—particularly Sharon Sandifer-Holmes, Bobbie Gallagher, and Cindy Schultz—thank you for letting me tell your stories and meet your remarkable children. You, and all parents raising and advocating for children with autism while somehow balancing the daily demands of life, are truly the world's unsung heroes. Finally, thank you to Crystal Yakacki, my editor at Seven Stories Press, who believed in this topic, entrusted me to write it, and provided such invaluable insight and guidance along the way. I'm honored to be part of such a phenomenal group of authors.

NOTES

❧

INTRODUCTION: THE MISSING PERCENTAGE

1. Robert Miller, "Hatters' lives remembered," *The News-Times*, February 1, 2011, http://www.newstimes.com/local/article/Hatters-lives-remembered-985616.php.
2. "Medical Management Guidelines for Mercury," Agency for Toxic Substances & Disease Registry, last updated March 3, 2011, accessed November 21, 2011, http://www.atsdr.cdc.gov/mmg/mmg.asp?id=106&tid=24.
3. "Mercury," Occupational Safety & Health Administration, United States Department of Labor, last updated October 4, 2007, accessed January 3, 2012, http://www.osha.gov/SLTC/mercury/index.html.
4. Catherine Rice, "Prevalence of Autism Spectrum Disorders—Autism and Developmental Disabilities Monitoring Network, United States, 2006," Centers for Disease Control and Prevention, *MMWR* 58, no. SS10 (December 2009): 9–20, http://www.cdc.gov/mmwr/preview/mmwrhtml/ss5810a1.htm.
5. Young Shin Kim, Bennett L. Leventhal, Yun-Joo Koh, Eric Fombonne, Eugene Laska, et al., "Prevalence of Autism Spectrum Disorders in a Total Population Sample, The American Journal of Psychiatry 168, no. 9 (September 2011); 904-912, http://ajp.psychiatryonline.org/article.aspx?articleid=116570.
6. Rice, "Prevalence of Autism Spectrum Disorders—Autism and Developmental Disabilities Monitoring Network, United States, 2006," Centers for Disease Control and Prevention, MMWR 58, no. SS10 (December2009):9-20, http://www.cdc.gov/mmwr/preview/mmwrhtml/ss5810a1.htm.
7. S. Bernard, A. Enayati, L. Redwood, H. Roger, and T. Binstock, "Autism: A Novel Form of Mercury Poisoning," *Medical Hypotheses* 56, no. 3 (April 2001): 462–471.
8. "What Are the Autism Spectrum Disorders?" National Institute of Mental Health, accessed October 5, 2011, http://www.nimh.nih.gov/health/publications/autism/what-are-the-autism-spectrum-disorders.shtml.
9. Alok Jha and Sarah Boseley, "Scientists Have the Genetic Causes of Autism in Their Sights," *The Guardian*, June 9, 2010, http://www.guardian.co.uk/science/2010/jun/09/autism-study-genetic-causes.
10. Dalila Pinto, Alistair T. Pagnamenta, Lambertus Klei, Richard Anney, Daniele Merico, et al., "Functional Impact of Global Rare Copy Number Variation in Autism Spectrum Disorders," Nature 466 (2010): 368–372, http://www.nature.com/nature/journal/v466/n7304/full/nature09146.html.
11. "Largest-Ever Search for Autism Genes Reveals New Clues," National Institute of Mental Health, February 18, 2007, http://www.nimh.nih.gov/science-news/2007/largest-ever-search-for-autism-genes-reveals-new-clues.shtml.

12. Nancy Shute, "To Help Cure Autism, Share Your DNA," U.S. News & World Report, June 9, 2010, http://health.usnews.com/health-news/blogs/onparenting/2010/06/09/to-help-cure-autism-share-your-dna.

13. Joachim Hallmayer, Sue Cleveland, Andrea Torres, et al., "Genetic Heritability and Shared Environmental Factors Among Twin Pairs with Autism," *Archives of General Psychiatry* 68, no. 11 (November 2011): 1095–1102.

14. Ibid.

15. Shuk-mei Ho, interview with the author, May 2010.

16. Ibid.

17. Marcus E. Pembrey, Lars Olov Bygren, Gunnar Kaati, et al., "Sex-specific, Male-line Transgenerational Responses in Humans," *European Journal of Human Genetics* 14 (2006): 159–166.

28. Hallmayer, "Genetic Heritability and Shared Environmental Factors Among Twin Pairs with Autism," 2011.

19. Michael Merzenich, interview with the author, October 8, 2009.

20. "Child Population: Number of Children (in Millions) Ages 0-17 in the United States by Age, 1950-2010 and Projected 2030-2050," Federal Interagency Forum on Child and Family Statistics, 2011, accessed November 21, 2011, http://www.childstats.gov/americaschildren/tables/pop1.asp?popup=true.

21. Rice, "Prevalence of Autism Spectrum Disorders—Autism and Developmental Disabilities Monitoring Network, United States, 2006," Centers for Disease Control and Prevention, MMWR 58, no. SS10 (December2009):9–20, http://www.cdc.gov/mmwr/preview/mmwrhtml/ss5810a1.htm.

22. "Facts About Autism," Autism Speaks, accessed May 11, 2011, http://www.autismspeaks.org/what-autism/facts-about-autism.

23. Irva Hertz-Picciotto, "Autism & Toxic Chemical Exposure: What is the Relationship?" (teleconference), Safer Chemicals, Healthy Families, June 7, 2011.

24. Gregory J. de Montfort and Rosemary Boon, "Stages of Brain Development," 2000, accessed June 8, 2011, sirricenter.com/pdfarticles/06_Stages_of_Brain_Development.pdf.

25. Margaret L. Bauman and Thomas L. Kemper, *The Neurobiology of Autism, 2nd ed.* (Baltimore: Johns Hopkins University Press, 2005).

26. Virginia Rauh, Robin Garfinkel, Frederica P. Perera, et al., "Impact of Prenatal Chlorpyrifos Exposure on Neurodevelopment in the First 3 Years of Life Among Inner-City Children," *Pediatrics* 118, no. 6 (December 2006): e1845–e1859.

27. C. M. Hultman, P. Sparen, S. Cnattingius, "Perinatal Risk Factors for Infantile Autism," *Epidemiology* 13, no. 4 (July 2002): 417–23.

28. Review of Exposure Data and Assessments for Select Dialkyl Ortho-Phthalates," Consumer Product Safety Commission, Feb. 24, 2010, http://www.cpsc.gov/about/cpsia/pthalexp.pdf.

29. DavidRose, "Lancet Journal Retracts Andrew Wakefield MMR Scare Paper," *The Times*, February 3, 2010.

30. "Timeline: Thimerosal in Vaccines (1999–2008)," Centers for Disease Control and Prevention. February 8, 2011, http://www.cdc.gov/vaccinesafety/concerns/thimerosal/thimerosal_timeline.html. Accessed November 3, 2011.

31. "Mercury in Vaccines is at Safe Levels, Study Suggests," University of Rochester Medical Center, December 2, 2002, http://www.urmc.rochester.edu/news/story/index.cfm?id=160.

32. "Mercury in Vaccines," Network for Immunization Information, last updated August 6, 2008, accessed January 11, 2012, http://www.immunizationinfo.org/issues/thimer-

osal-mercury/mercury-vaccines.

33. Ibid.
34. "About the NTP," National Toxicology Program, last updated February 17, 2005, accessed November 23, 2011, http://ntp.niehs.nih.gov/?objectid=7201637B-BDB7-CEBA-F57E39896A08F1BB.
35. "HPV Chemical Hazard Data Availability Study," US Environmental Protection Agency, last updated Aug. 2, 2010, accessed Jan. 4, 2012, http://www.epa.gov/hpv/pubs/general/hazchem.htm.
36. "Green Cleaning Supplies," Sierra Club, accessed October 14, 2011, http://www.sierraclubgreenhome.com/go-green/cleaning/green-household-cleaning/.
37. "About the NTP," National Toxicology Program, accessed November 23, 2011.
38. "Introduction to Biomonitoring Topics," *America's Children and the Environment*, 3rd Edition (draft), US Environmental Protection Agency, last updated April 22, 2011, accessed November 21, 2011, www.epa.gov/ace/ace3draft/draft_pdfs/biomonitoring_intro.pdf.
39. "National Report on Human Exposure to Environmental Chemicals (Fourth Report)," Centers for Disease Control and Prevention, February 2011, accessed June 9, 2011, www.cdc.gov/exposurereport.
40. "Body Burden—The Pollution in Newborns," Environmental Working Group, July 14, 2005, http://www.ewg.org/reports/bodyburden2/execsumm.php.
41. Sonya Lunder, Renee Sharp, Amy Ling, and Caroline Colesworthy, "Toxic Fire Retardants (PBDEs) in Human Breast Milk," Environmental Working Group, September 2003, http://www.ewg.org/reports/mothersmilk#.Tprky3Kvl2I.
42. "Body Burden—The Pollution in Newborns," Environmental Working Group, July 14, 2005, http://www.ewg.org/reports/bodyburden2/execsumm.php.
43. Lisa A. Croen, Judith K. Grether, Cathleen Yoshida, Roxana Odouli, and Victoria Hendrick, "Antidepressant Use During Pregnancy and Childhood Autism Spectrum Disorders," Archives of General Psychiatry 68, no. 11 (Nov. 2011): 1104-1112, http://archpsyc.ama-assn.org/cgi/content/short/68/11/1104.
44. Eric Hollander, ed., Austism Spectrum Disorders (New York: Marcel Dekker, Inc., 2005).
45. Centers for Disease "Blood Lead Levels in Young Children—United States and Selected Statees, 1996–1999," Morbidity and Mortality Weekly Report 49, no. 50 (December 22, 2000): 1133-7, http://www.cdc.gov/mmwr/preview/mmwrhtml/mm4950a3.htm.
46. Philip J. Landrigan, "Greening Our Children" (conference), Hyatt Regency Greenwich, May 9, 2011.

CHAPTER ONE: UNCOUNTED NUMBERS

1. "Mercury in Canned Tuna Still a Concern," Consumer Reports, last updated January 2011, access January 19, 2012, http://www.consumerreports.org/cro/magazine-archive/2011/january/food/mercury-in-tuna/overview/index.htm.
2. Gloria B. Ramirez, Olive Pagulayan, Hirokatsu Akagi, et al., "Tagum Study II: Follow-up Study at Two Years of Age After Prenatal Exposure to Mercury," *Pediatrics* 111, no. 3 (March 2003): e289–e295.
3. Gloria B. Ramirez, Cristina Vince Cruz, Olive Pagulayan, Enrique Ostrea, and Crispin Dalisay, "The Tagum Study I: Analysis and Clinical Correlates of Mercury in Maternal and Cord Blood, Breast Milk, Meconium and Infants' Hair," *Pediatrics*, 106, no. 4 (October 2000): 774–781.

4. Fei Xue, Claudia Holzman, Mohammad Hossein Rahbar, Kay Trosko, Lawrence Fischer, "Maternal Fish Consumption, Mercury Levels, and Risk of Preterm Delivery," *Environmental Health Perspectives* 115, no. 1 (January 2007):42–47.

5. Christopher Fisher, "Low Birthweight Infants Have Five Times Rate of Autism," *The Behavioral Medicine Report*, October 17, 2011, http://www.bmedreport.com/archives/31385.

6. "What You Need to Know About Mercury in Fish and Shellfish," US Food and Drug Administration, 2004.

7. Jun Ui, ed., Industrial Pollution in Japan (Tokyo: United Nations University Press, 1992).

8. "Frequently Asked Questions—Minamata Disease Q&A," National Institute for Minamata Disease, accessed June 10, 2011, http://www.nimd.go.jp/archives/english/tenji/e_corner/etop.html.

9. Hiroko Nakata, "Koizumi Issues Official Minamata Apology," *The Japan Times*, April 29, 2006.

10. Michael Brauer, Cornel Lencar, Lillian Tamburic, Mieke Koehoorn, Paul Demers and Catherine Karr, "A Cohort Study of Traffic-Related Air Pollution Impacts on Birth Outcomes," Environmental Health Perspectives 116, no. 5 (May 2008): 680–686, http://www.ncbi.nlm.nih.gov/pmc/articles/PMC2367679/?too l=pubmed.

11. "CHE Toxicant and Disease Database," The Collaborative on Health and the Environment, accessed May 8, 2011, http://www.healthandenvironment.org/tddb.

12. Mark Mitchell, interview with the author, July 14, 2010.

13. M. Briacombe, X. Ming, and M. Lamendola, "Prenatal and Birth Complications in Autism," Maternal and Child Health Journal 11, no. 1 (2007): 73–79

14. Sharon Sandifer-Holmes, interview with the author, June 6, 2010.

15. "Bridgeport Harbor Station," SourceWatch, last modified June 12, 2011, accessed November 23, 2011, www.sourcewatch.org/index.php?title=Bridgeport_Harbor_Station.

16. "NAACP Cleaning the Air Road Tour," Sourcewatch, April 2012, http://www.sourcewatch.org/index.php?title=Bridgeport_Harbor_Station#Emissions_Data.

17. "BGreen 2020: A Sustainability Plan for Bridgeport, Connecticut," City of Bridgeport and Bridgeport Regional Business Council, March 5, 2010, http://www.rpa.org/2010/03/bgreen-2020-a-sustainability-plan-for-bridgeport-connecticut.html.

18. "A Review, by State, of Operating Municipal Solid Waste Incinerators, #5: California to Bristol, Connecticut," World on Waste USA, Inc., December 1993–January 1994, http://www.americanhealthstudies.org/wastenot/wn255.htm.

19. Mark Mitchell, interview with the author, July 14, 2010.

20. Keila Torres, "GE's Plans to Take Down Massive Factory Complex Stalls," *Connecticut Post*, July 3, 2010, http://www.ctpost.com/local/article/GE-s-plans-to-take-down-massive-factory-complex-564554.php.

21. Ray Bendici, "Remington Arms, Bridgeport," Damned Connecticut, accessed July 15, 2011, www.damnedct.com/remington-arms-bridgeport.

22. Denis J. O'Malley III, "Small Steps on Long Road to Cleaning Up GE Property," *Connecticut Post*, September 5, 2009, http://www.ctpost.com/news/article/Small-steps-on-long-road-to-cleaning-up-GE-26057.php.

23. Gayle C. Windham, Lixia Zhang, Robert Gunier, Lisa A Croen, and Judith K. Grether, "Autism Spectrum Disorders in Relation to Distribution of Hazardous Air Pollutants in the San Francisco Bay Area," Environmental Health Perspectives 114, no. 9 (September 2006): 1438–1444, http://www.ncbi.nlm.nih.gov/pmc/articles/PMC1570060/.

24. "Priority List of Hazardous Substances," Agency for Toxic Substances & Disease Registry, last updated October 25, 2011, accessed November 21, 2011, http://www.atsdr. cdc.gov/SPL/index.html.

25. Windham, Zhang, Gunier, Croen, and Grether, "Autism Spectrum Disorders in Relation to Distribution of Hazardous Air Pollutants in the San Francisco Bay Area," Environmental Health Perspectives, 2006.

26. Raymond F. Palmer, S. Blanchard, and R. Wood, "Proximity to Point Sources of Environmental Mercury Release as a Predictor of Autism Prevalence," Health Place 15, no.1 (March 2009): 18–24.

27. Ibid.

28. J. Felix Rogers and Anne L. Dunlop, "Air Pollution and Very Low Birth Weight Infants: A Target Population?" Pediatrics 118, no. 1 (July 2006):156–164.

29. Patricia O'Campo, Jessica G. Burke, Jennifer Culhane, et al., "Neighborhood Deprivation and Preterm Birth Among Non-Hispanic Black and White Women in Eight Geographic Areas in the United States," American Journal of Epidemiology 167, no. 2 (January 2008): 155–163.

30. Patricia O'Campo, interview with the author, July 20, 2010.

31. Laura R. Ment and Betty R. Vohr, "Preterm Birth and the Developing Brain," The Lancet Neurology 7, no. 5 (May 2008): 378–379.

32. Rice, "Prevalence of Autism Spectrum Disorders—Autism and Developmental Disabilities Monitoring Network, United States, 2006," 2009.

33. Mitchell, interview with the author, 2010.

34. "Bridgeport (city), Connecticut," State & County QuickFacts, last updated December 23, 2011, accessed January 14, 2012, http://quickfacts.census.gov/qfd/states/09/0908000.html.

35. "Best Places to Live 2006," CNN Money, accessed November 23, 2011, http://money.cnn.com/magazines/moneymag/bplive/2006/index.html.

36. "Release Reports," TRI Explorer, US Environmental Protection Agency, last updated November 23, 2011, accessed November 23, 2011, http://iaspub.epa.gov/triexplorer/tri_release.chemical.

37. "Getting the Big Picture on Houston's Air Pollution," NASA, last updated November 30, 2007, accessed November 23, 2011, http://www.nasa.gov/vision/earth/everydaylife/archives/HP_ILP_Feature_03.html.

38. "Half of Americans Still Affected by Dangerous Pollution Levels," American Lung Association, May 2, 2011, http://www.citymayors.com/environment/polluted_uscities.html.

39. Sandifer-Holmes, interview with the author, 2010.

40. D. S. Mandell, J. Listerud, E. E. Levy and J. A. Pinto-martin, "Race Difference in the Age at Diagnosis Among Medicaide-eligible Children with Autism," Journal of the American Academy of Child Adolescent Psychiatry 41, no. 12 (December 2002): 14447–53, http://www.ncbi.nlm.nih.gov/pubmed/12447031.

41. David S. Mandell, Richard F. Ittenbach, Susan E. Levy, and Jennifer A. Pinto-Martin, "Disparities in Diagnosis Received Prior to a Diagnosis of Autism Spectrum Disorder," Journal of Autism and Developmental Disorders 37, no. 9 (October 2007): 1795–1802.

42. "Learn the Signs. Act Early," Centers for Disease Control and Prevention, last updated October 1, 2010, accessed November 22, 2011, http://www.cdc.gov/ncbddd/actearly/index.html.

43. "Special Education," Education Week, last updated July 7, 2011, accessed January 5, 2012, http://www.edweek.org/ew/issues/special-education/.

44.   Kathleen Megan, "Parents, Advocates Seek More Prompt Diagnosis of Minority Children," *The Hartford Courant*, May 14, 2007, http://articles.courant.com/2007-05-14/features/0705140504_1_autism-and-race-autism-spectrum-disorders-developmental-disorder.

45.   Crystal Phend, "No Environmental Link in California Autism Clusters," *MedPage Today*, January 6, 2010, http://www.medpagetoday.com/Neurology/Autism/17832.

46.   Ka-Yuet Liu, Marissa King, and Peter S. Bearman, "Social Influence and the Autism Epidemic," *American Journal of Sociology* 115, no. 5 (March 2010): 1387–1434.

47.   Catherine Rice, "Prevalence of Autism Spectrum Disorders—Autism and Disabilities Monitoring Network, Six Sites, United States, 2000" Centers for Disease Control and Prevention, MMWR 56, no. SS01 (February 2007): 1–11, http://www.cdc.gov/mmwr/preview/mmwrhtml/ss5601a1.htm.

48.   Young Shin Kim, Bennett L. Leventhal, Yun-Joo Koh, Eric Fombonne, Eugene Laska, et al., "Prevalence of Autism Spectrum Disorders in a Total Population Sample, The American Journal of Psychiatry 168, no. 9 (Spetember 2011): 904–912, http://ajp.psychiatryonline.org/article.aspx?articleid=116570.

49.   Jon Hamilton, "Study Suggests Autism Rate May Be Underestimated," NPR, last updated May 9, 2011, accessed January 5, 2012, http://www.npr.org/2011/05/09/136066097/autism-may-be-far-more-commonstudy- suggests.

50.   D.V. Keen, F. D. Reid, and D. Arnone, "Autism, Ethnicity and Maternal Immigration," *The British Journal of Psychiatry* 196, no. 4 (April 2010): 274–281.

51.   Ibid.

CHAPTER TWO: FOREIGN BODIES

1.   "Public Health Statement for Mercury," Agency for Toxic Substances & Disease Registry, March 1999, http://www.atsdr.cdc.gov/phs/phs.asp?id=112&tid=24#bookmark04.

2.   Ibid.

3.   Ibid.

4.   Richard E. Besser, "Children's Exposure to Elemental Mercury: A National Review of Exposure Events," Agency for Toxic Substances & Disease Registry and Centers for Disease Control and Prevention Mercury Workgroup, February 2009, www.atsdr.cdc.gov/mercury/docs/MercuryRTCFinal2013345.pdf.

5.   Ibid.

6.   Eric Yates and Robert Frey, "Health Consultation: Mercury Exposures from 3M Tartan Brand Floors," Agency for Toxic Substances & Disease Registry, last updated December 15, 2009, accessed November 23, 2011, http://www.atsdr.cdc.gov/hac/pha/pha.asp?docid=664&pg=1.

7.   Ibid.

8.   Helen V. Ratajczak, "Theoretical Aspects of Autism: Causes—A Review," Journal of Immunotoxicology 8, no. 1 (2011):68–79, http://www.cogforlife.org/ratajczakstudy.pdf.

9.   "Mercury in New Jersey Day-Care Center 3,000 Times Standard," Public Employees for Environmental Responsibility, February 11, 2008, http://www.peer.org/news/news_id.php?row_id=987.

10.   Jan Hefler, "Kiddie Kollege Owners, Parents Settle Suit Over Tots' Exposure to Toxin for $1 million," *The Inquirer*, October 20, 2010, http://articles.philly.com/2010-10-20/news/24983418_1_mercury-exposure-day-care-operators-sullivans.

11.   "Mercury in New Jersey Day-Care Center 3,000 Times Standard," Public Employees for Environmental Responsibility, 2008.

12. Besser, "Children's Exposure to Elemental Mercury: A National Review of Exposure Events," 2009.

13. Ibid.

14. "Epidemiologic Notes and Reports Elemental Mercury Poisoning in a Household—Ohio, 1989," Centers for Disease Control and Prevention, *MMWR* 39, no. 25 (June 1990):424-425, www.cdc.gov/mmwr/preview/mmwrhtml/00001652.htm.

15. Helen V. Ratajczak, "Theoretical Aspects of Autism: Causes—A Review," Journal of Immunotoxicology 8, no. 1 (2011):68–79, http://www.cogforlife.org/ratajczakstudy. pdf.

16. "Public Health Statement for Mercury," Agency for Toxic Substances & Disease Registry, March 1999, http://www.atsdr.cdc.gov/PHS/PHS .asp?id=112&tid=24.

17. Dan R. Laks, "Assessment of Chronic Mercury Exposure Within the US Population, National Health and Nutrition Examination Survey, 1999-2006," *Biometals* 22, no. 6 (December 2009): 1103–1114.

18. E. J. Mundell, "Blood Mercury Levels Rising Among US Women," ABC News, August 25, 2009, http://abcnews.go.com/Health/Healthday/story?id=8401245.

19. "Body Burden—The Pollution in Newborns," Environmental Working Group, July 14, 2005, http://www.ewg.org/reports/bodyburden2/execsumm.php.

20. James B. Adams, J. Romdalvik, V.M. Ramanujam, and M. S. Legator, "Mercury, Lead, and Zinc in Baby Teeth of Children with Autism Versus Controls," *Journal of Toxicology and Environmental Health* 70, no. 12 (June 2007): 1046–1051.

21. James B. Adams, interview with the author, October 10, 2009.

22. James B. Adams, J. Romdalvik, K.E. Levine, and L. Hu, "Mercury in First-Cut Baby Hair of Children with Autism Versus Typically-Developing Children," *Toxicological and Environmental Chemistry* 90, no. 4 (July–August 2008): 739–753.

23. R. Rowland, R. D. Robinson, and R. A. Doherty, "Effects of Diet on Mercury Metabolism and Excretion in Mice Given Methymercury: Role of Gut Flora," Archives of Environmental Health 39, no. 6 (November 1984): 401–8, http://www.ncbi.nlm.nih. gov/pubmed/6524959.

24. Adams, interview with the author, 2009.

25. "Basic Information: Mercury," US Environmental Protection Agency, last updated October 1, 2010, accessed November 23, 2011, http://www.epa.gov/hg/about.htm.

26. "National Lake Fish Tissue Study," US Environmental Protection Agency, last updated September 29, 2011, accessed November 23, 2011, www.epa.gov/waterscience/ fishstudy.

27. "National Listing of Fish Advisories 2008," US Environmental Protection Agency, last updated November 1, 2011, accessed November 23, 2011, http://water.epa.gov/ scitech/swguidance/fishshellfish/fishadvisories/fs2008.cfm.

28. Emily Fisher, "A Big Win for Safer Seafood," Oceana.org, last updated December 10, 2010, accessed January 16, 2012, http://na.oceana.org/en/blog/2010/12/a-big-win-for-safer-seafood.

29. "August 2006 Fact Sheet: National Vehicle Mercury Switch Recovery Program," US Environmental Protection Agency, last updated October 1, 2010, accessed November 23, 2011, http://www.epa.gov/hg/switchfs.htm.

30. "Texas Coal Plant's 50,000 Air Pollution Violations Lead to Legal Challenge," Earthjustice, last updated September 2, 2010, accessed January 16, 2012, http:// earthjustice.org/news/press/2010/texas-coal-plant-s-50-000-air-pollution-violations-lead-to-legal-challenge.

31. "Dirty Kilowatts: America's Top Fifty Power Plant Mercury Polluters," Environmen-

tal Integrity Project, March 2010, http://www.environmentalintegrity.org/news_reports/documents/DirtyKilowatts-Top50MercuryPowerPlantReport.pdf.

32. R. F. Palmer, S. Blanchard, Z. Stein, D. Mandekk, and C. Miller, "Environmental Mercury Release, Special Education Rates, and Autism Disorder: An Ecological Study of Texas," Health Place 12, no. 4 (December 2006): 749–50, http://www.ncbi.nlm.nih.gov/pubmed/16338635.

33. "Map of Texas," US Energy Information Administration, last updated October 2009, accessed November 23, 2011, http://www.eia.gov/state/state-energy-profiles.cfm?sid=TX.

34. Jeff Sell, interview with the author, May 25, 2010.

35. "Toxicological Profile for Benzene," US Department of Health and Human Services, Agency for Toxic Substances & Disease Registry, August 2007, http://www.atsdr.cdc.gov/toxprofiles/tp3.pdf.

36. "Participant Body Burdens," Mind, Disrupted, accessed November 23, 2011, http://www.minddisrupted.org/findings.participant.php.

37. Ibid.

38. Jeff Sell, interview with the author, May 25, 2010.

39. Hertz-Picciotto, "Autism & Toxic Chemical Exposure: What is the Relationship?" 2011.

40. "Fact Sheet: Triclosan," National Report on Human Exposure to Environmental Chemicals," last updated February 28, 2011, accessed January 16, 2012, http://www.cdc.gov/exposurereport/Triclosan_FactSheet.html.

41. "Exposure In Utero to Diethylstilbestrol and Related Synthetic Hormones: Association With Vaginal and Cervical Cancers and Other Abnormalities," National Cancer Institute, *Journal of the American Medical Association*, 236, no. 10 (September 1976): 1107–1109.

42. "Prenatal Origins of Endocrine Disruption: Introduction," The Endocrine Disruption Exchange, accessed November 23, 2011, http://www.endocrinedisruption.com/prenatal.introduction.php.

43. Jonathan Chevrier, Kim G. Harley, Asa Bradman, Myrian Gharbi, Andreas Sjodin, and Brenda Eskenazi, "Polybrominated Diphenyl Ether (PBDE) Flame Retardents and Thyroid Hormone During Pregnancy," Envrionmental Health Perspectives 118, no. 10 (October 2012), http://ehp03.niehs.nih.gov/article/info%3Adoi%2F10.1289%2Fehp.1001905.

44. V. J. Pop, J. L. Kuijpens, A. L. van Baar, et al., "Low Maternal Free Thyroxine Concentrations During Early Pregnancy are Associated with Impaired Psychomotor Development in Infancy," *Clinical Endocrinology* 50, no. 2 (February 1999): 149–155.

45. Hertz-Picciotto, "Autism & Toxic Chemical Exposure: What is the Relationship?" 2011.

46. "Polybrominated Diphenylethers (PBDEs)," US Environmental Protection Agency, last updated January 26, 2010, accessed November 23, 2011, http://www.epa.gov/opptintr/pbde/.

47. Fourth Report on Human Exposure to Environmental Chemicals," Department of Health and Human Services, Centers for Disease Control and Prevention, 2009, accessed January 16, 2012, http://www.cdc.gov/exposurereport/pdf/FourthReport.pdf.

48. Julie B. Herbstman, Andreas Sjodin, Matthew Kurzon, et al., "Prenatal Exposure to PBDEs and Neurodevelopment," *Environmental Health Perspectives* 118, no. 5 (January 2010): 712–719, http://www.greensciencepolicy.org/sites/default/files/HerbstmanEHP2010%20PBDEs%20and%20neuro%20imparment14.pdf.

49. D. Merionyte, K. Noren, A. Bergman, "Analysis of Polybrominate Diphenyl Ethers in

Swedish Human Milk. A Time-related Trend Study, 1972–1997," Journal of Toxicology and Environmental Health, Part A 58, no. 6 (November 1999):329–41, http://www.ncbi.nlm.nih.gov/pubmed/10580757.

50. "Chemicals: PDBEs," Healthy Milk, Healthy Baby, Natural Resources Defense Council, last modified March 25, 2005, accessed November 23, 2011, http://www.nrdc.org/breastmilk/pbde.asp.

51. Arnold Schecter, Marian Pavuk, Olaf Papke, John Jake Ryan, Linda Birnbaum, and Robin Rosen, "Polybrominated Diphenyl Ethers (PBDEs) in US Mothers' Milk," Environmental Health Perspectives 111, no. 14 (November 2003): 1723–1729, http://ehp03.niehs.nih.gov/article/info%3Adoi%2F10.1289%2Fehp.6466.

52. Suruchi Chandra, "Autism & Toxic Chemical Exposure: What is the Relationship?" (teleconference), Safer Chemicals Healthy Families, June 7, 2011.

53. Ibid.

54. "Mind, Disrupted: How Toxic Chemicals May Change How We Think and Who We Are," Mind, Disrupted, accessed November 23, 2011, http://www.minddisrupted.org/documents/Mind%20Disrupted%20Summary.pdf.

CHAPTER THREE: DUMPED ON

1. "French's Landfill," Township of Brick New Jersey, accessed November 25, 2011, http://www.twp.brick.nj.us/content.asp?ContentId=569.

2. "EPA proposed Cleanup Plan for Brick Township Landfille Superfund Site," United States Environmental Protection Agency, last updated September 4, 2008, accessed January 16, 2012, http://yosemite.epa.gov/opa/admpress.nsf/0/8F878C9A9D9E826 3852574BA00623533.

3. "Brick Township Landfill Superfund Site," US Environmental Protection Agency, July 2008, http://www.epa.gov/region2/superfund/npl/bricktownship/bricktownship_proposedplan.pdf.

4. Bobbie Gallagher, interview with the author, April 3, 2010.

5. Samuel M. Goldman, Patricia J. Quinlan, G. Webster Ross, Connie Marras, Cheryl Meng, Grace S. Bhudhikanok, Kathleen Comyns, et al., "Solvent Exposures and Parkinson Disease Risk in Twins," Annals of Neurology, published online November 14, 2011, http://onlinelibrary.wiley.com/doi/10.1002/ana.22629/abstract.

6. LC Backer, DL Ashley, MA Bonin, GL Cardinali, et al., "Household Exposures to Drinking Water Disinfection By-products; Whole Blood Trihalomethane Levels," Journal of Exposure Science and Environmental Epidemiology 10 (2002): 321–326.

7. Marshalyn Yeargin-Allsopp, Catherine Rice, Tanya Karapurkar, nancy Doernberg, Coleen Boyle, and Catherine Murphy, "Prevalence of Autism in US Metropolitan Area," Journal of the American Medical Association 289, no. 1 (January 1, 2003): 49–55, http://jama.ama-assn.org/content/289/1/49.full.pdf.

8. "Case-control Study of Childhood Cancers in Dover Township (Ocean County), New Jersey," Division of Epidemiology, Environmental and Occupational Health, New Jersey Department of Health and Senior Services and Agency for Toxic Substances & Disease Registry, December 2001, http://rarediseases.about.com/gi/o.htm?zi=1/XJ&zTi=1&sdn=rarediseases&cdn=health&tm=63&f=10&su=p284.9.336.ip_p736.9.336.ip_&tt=2&bt=0&bts=0&zu=http%3A//www.state.nj.us/health/eoh/hhazweb/case-control_pdf/Volume_I/Voli.pdf.

9. "Toms River Homeowners Reach $20M Settlement with Chemical Company Accused of Dumping Toxic Waste," The Associated Press, June 14, 2011, http://www.nj.com/news/index.ssf/2011/06/toms_river_homeowners_reach_20.html.

10. "Public Health Assessment, Brick Township Investigation, Brick Township, Ocean County, New Jersey," Superfund Site Assessment Branch, Division of Health Assessment and Consultation, Agency for Toxic Substances & Disease Registry, 2000, http://www.atsdr.cdc.gov/hac/pha/bri/bri_toc.html.

11. "Brick Township Landfill Superfund Site," 2008.

12. Sanford Lewis, Brian Keating, Dick Russell, Cathy Hinds, ed., and Linda King, ed., "Inconclusive By Design: Waste, Fraud and Abuse in Federal Environmental Health Research," Environmental Health Network and the National Toxics Campaign Fund, May 1992, http://www.ejnet.org/toxics/inconclusive.pdf.

13. "Living Near Hazardous Waste Sites," US Environmental Protection Agency, last updated October 12, 2010, accessed November 25, 2011, http://www.epa.gov/Region2/health/superfund-sites.htm.

14. Barry L. Johnson, "A Review of the Effects of Hazardous Waste on Reproductive Health," *American Journal of Obstetric Gynecology* 181, no. 1 (July 1999): S12–S16, http://www.columbia.edu/itc/hs/pubhealth/windgasse/client_edit/hw-obgyn.pdf.

15. "QuickStats: Spina Bifada and Anencephaly Rates—United States, 1991, 1995, 2000, and 2005," MMRW Weekly 57, no. 1 (January 11, 2008): 15, http://www.cdc.gov/mmwr/preview/mmwrhtml/mm57o1a7.htm.

16. Joyce A. Martin, Brady E. Hamilton, Paul D, Sutton, Stephanie J. Ventura, Fay Menacker, Sharon Kirmeyer, and Martha L. Munson, "Births: Final Data for 2005," National Vital Statistics Reports 56, no. 6 (December 5, 2007), http://www.cdc.gov/nchs/data/nvsr/nvsr56/nvsr56_06.pdf.

17. K. Stromland, V. Nordin, M. Miller, B. Akerstron, C. Gillberg, "Autism in Thalidomide Embryopathy. A Population Study," Developmental Medicine & Child Neurology 36 (1994): 351–356.

18. Neil Vargesson, "Thalidomide-induced Limb Defects: Resolving a 50-Year-Old Puzzle," Biological Sciences 31, no. 12 (2009): 1327–1336, http://www.mendeley.com/research/thalidomideinduced-limb-defects-resolving-50yearold-puzzle/#.

19. Patricia M. Rodier, Jennifer L. Ingram, Barbara Tisdale, Sarah Nelson, and John Romano, "Embryological Origin for Autism: Developmental Anomalies of the Cranial Nerve Motor Nuclei," *The Journal of Comparative Neurology* 370, no. 2 (June 1996): 247–261.

20. Ibid.

21. "Public Health Assessment, Brick Township Investigation, Brick Township, Ocean County, New Jersey," 2000.

22. Carol Reinisch, interview with the author, July 30, 2010.

23. "Pollutant Mixes Can Affect Nerve Cell Growth," Marine Biological Laboratory *LabNotes* 15, no. 1 (Spring 2005), http://www.mbl.edu/publications/labnotes/2005/05_spring02.html.

24. Carol Reinisch, interview with the author, July 30, 2010.

25. Jill Kreiling, interview with the author, August 5, 2010.

26. Sara Rose Guariglia, "Gender Specific Changes in Key Regulators of Neurodevelopment and Autistic Behavioral Pathology in Mice Exposed to Water Chlorination Byproducts," (PhD dissertation, City University of New York, 2010).

27. "National Priorities List," US Environmental Protection Agency, last updated December 22, 2011, accessed January 16, 2012, http://www.epa.gov/superfund/sites/npl/index.htm.

28. "New Jersey Sites," US Environmental Protection Agency, last updated October 12, 2011, accessed January 16, 2012, http://www.epa.gov/region02/cleanup/sites/njtoc_name.htm.

29. "Statement of Senator Barbara Boxer," Environment and Public Works Committee Oversight Hearing on the Superfund Program, June 15, 2006, http://epw.senate. gov/109th/Boxer_Statement.pdf.

30. "EPA Adds 10 Hazardous Waste Sites to the Superfund's National Priority List," US Environmental Protection Agency, March 8, 2011, http://www.epa.gov/aging/press/ epanews/2011/2011_0308_1.htm.

31. "Cleanup Process," US Environmental Protection Agency, last updated August 9, 2011, accessed January 16, 2012, http://epa.gov/superfund/cleanup/index.htm.

32. Catherine Rice, "Prevalence of Autism Spectrum Disorders—Autism and Disabilities Monitoring Network, Six Sites, United States, 2000" Centers for Disease Control and Prevention, MMWR 56, no. SS01 (February 2007): 1–11, http://www.cdc.gov/ mmwr/preview/mmwrhtml/ss5601a1.htm.

33. "I-Team: Possible Autism 'Cluster' Concerns Mothers," WBALTV, last updated July 7, 2009, accessed November 25, 2011, http://www.wbaltv.com/r/19969446/detail. html.

34. "TRI On-site and Off-site Reported Disposed of or Otherwise Released (in pounds), for facilities in All Industries, for All Chemicals, Virginia, 2009," US Environmental Protection Agency TRI Explorer, last updated February 2010, accessed November 25, 2011, http://www.epa.gov/cgibin/broker?view=STFA&trilib=TRI Q1&sort=_VIEW_&sort_fmt=1&state=51&county=All+counties&chemical=_ ALL_&industry=ALL&year=2009&tab_rpt=1&fld=RELLBY&fld=TSFDSP&_ service=oiaa&_program=xp_tri.sasmacr.tristart.macro.

35. Alistair I. Clark, Alun E. McIntyre, Roger Perry, and John N. Lester, "Air Quality Measurement in the Vicinity of Airports," *Environmental Pollution Series B, Chemical and Physical* 6, no. 4 (1983): 245–261, http://www.sciencedirect.com/science/article/ pii/0143148X83900125.

36. Lawrence D. Rosen, "St. Anthony's Project," The Deirdre Imus Environmental Center for Pediatric Oncology, April 3, 2008, http://www.dienviro.com/s950/images/ st._anthony_s_project_summary_update_april08.pdf.

37. US Environmental Protection Agency, letter to David Michelman, April 15, 2009, http://yosemite.epa.gov/OA/RHC/EPAAdmin.nsf/Filings/73B27DE4ABA110F18 5257650004006oC/$File/Flexabar.CAFO.pdf.

38. "Specific Potential Contaminant Source Inventory," New Jersey Department of Environmental Protection, October 5, 2004, http://www.state.nj.us/dep/swap/reports/ appendixa_attachment2_0238001.pdf.

39. "Toxic Substances Portal—Tricholorethylene (TCE)," Agency for Toxic Substances & Disease Registry, last updated March 3, 2011, accessed November 25, 2011, http:// www.atsdr.cdc.gov/toxfaqs/tf.asp?id=172&tid=30.

40. "School Siting Guidelines," US Environmental Protection Agency, last updated October 2, 2011, accessed November 25, 2011, http://www.epa.gov/schools/siting/.

41. "Building Schools on Brownfields: Lessons Learned From California," The Bureau of National Affairs' Environmental Due Diligence Guide, no. 157, 2005, http://www. cpeo.org/pubs/BFschools.pdf.

42. Stephenie Hendricks, interview with the author, May 2010.

43. "Autism Study Looks at Pregnant Moms," WBALTV, March 22, 2011, http://www. wbaltv.com/r/27284567/detail.html.

CHAPTER FOUR: GUT REACTIONS

1. "Regressive Autism Is Real, Study Shows," *UW Today* (University of Washington),

August 4, 2005, http://www.washington.edu/news/archive/uweek/18670.
2. Gary D. Vogin, "Regressive Autism May Be Linked to Autoimmune Enteropathy," Medscape, April 30, 2002, http://www.medscape.com/viewarticle/432692.
3. Thomas L. Lowe, Kay Tanaka, Margretta R. Seashore, J. Gerald Young, and Donald Cohen, "Detection of Phenylketonuria in Autistic and Psychotic Children," Journal of the American Medical Association 243 (1980): 126–128, http://jama.ama-assn.org/content/243/2/126.full.pdf+html.
4. Cindy Schultz, interview with the author, June 12, 2010.
5. "Environmental Release Report: Oak Creek Power Plant," Scorecard, 2002, http://scorecard.goodguide.com/env-releases/facility.tcl?tri_id=53154KCRKP4801E#major_chemical_releases.
6. Thomas Content, "We Energies to Power Up as Demand for Energy Drops," The Journal Sentinel, January 25, 2010, http://www.jsonline.com/news/milwaukee/82567142.html.
7. "Oak Creek Site," Envirofacts, US Environmental Protection Agency Envirofacts, last updated November 26, 2011, accessed November 26, 2011, http://oaspub.epa.gov/enviro/multisys2.get_list_tri?tri_fac_id=53154KCRKP4801E.
8. "Scorecard's Noncancer Risk Scores," Scorecard, accessed November 25, 2011, http://scorecard.goodguide.com/env-releases/def/tep_noncancer.html.
9. "Pollution Locater: Facilities Contributing to Noncancer Hazards," Scorecard, accessed November 25, 2011, http://scorecard.goodguide.com/env-releases/county-facility-ranks.tcl?fips_county_code=55079&type=tep&category=noncancer&modifier=NA.
10. "Molybdenum—Mo," Lenntech, accessed November 25, 2011, http://www.lenntech.com/periodic/elements/mo.htm.
11. Christine Won, "Well Water Near Power Plant Contaminated: We Energies Supplying Bottled Water to Affected Residents While Seeking Source," The Journal Times, June 26, 2010, http://www.journaltimes.com/news/local/article_8df64c80-8197-11df-90a9-001cc4c03286.html.
12. Carol M. Ostrom, "More Parents Resisting Vaccines for Kids," The Seattle Times, July 16, 2006, http://seattletimes.nwsource.com/html/health/2003130272_resisters16m.html.
13. Darold A. Treffert, "Autistic Disorder: 52 Years Later: Some Common Sense Conclusions," Wisconsin Medical Society, 2011, http://www.wisconsinmedicalsociety.org/savant_syndrome/savant_articles/autistic_disorder.
14. J. B. Adams, J. Romdalvik. K. E. :Evine, and Lin-Wen Hu, "Mercury in First-Cut Baby Hair of Children with Autism Versus Typically-Developing Children," Toxicological & Envrironmental Chemistry 90, no. 4 (July 2008): 739–753.
15. "Healthy Milk, Healthy Baby," Natural Resources Defense Council, last modified May 22, 2001, accessed November 25, 2011, http://www.nrdc.org/breastmilk/chem13.asp.
16. J. B. Adams, J. Romdalvik. K. E. :Evine, and Lin-Wen Hu, "Mercury in First-Cut Baby Hair of Children with Autism Versus Typically-Developing Children," Toxicological & Envrironmental Chemistry 90, no. 4 (July 2008): 739–753.
17. Ibid.
18. "Is There a Link Between Autism and the Gut?" Massachusetts General Hospital, January 19, 2010, http://www.massgeneral.org/about/newsarticle.aspx?id=2043.
19. B. Sandhu, C. Steer, J. Golding, and A. Emond, "The Early Stool Patterns of Young Children with Autistic Spectrum Disorder," Archives of Disease in Childhood 94, no. 7 (March 2009): 497–500.

20. Brian Deer, "Wakefied's 'Autistic Enterocolitis' Under the Microscope," *British Medical Journal* 340 (April 2010): c1127.

21. Frank J. Kelly, "Oxidative Stress: It's Role in the Air Pollution and Adverse Health Effects," Occupational and Environmental Medicine 60, no. 8 (2003): 612–616, http://oem.bmj.com/content/60/8/612.full.

22. S. Jill James, Paul Cutler, Stepan Melnyk, et al., "Metabolic Biomarkers of Increased Oxidative Stress and Impaired Methylation Capacity in Children with Autism," *The American Journal of Clinical Nutrition* 80, no. 6 (December 2004): 1611–1617, http://www.ajcn.org/content/80/6/1611.full.

23. S. Jill James, interview with the author, April 8, 2010.

24. Shauna Layton, interview with the author, October 23, 2009.

25. Kenneth Bock, interview with the author, October 12, 2009.

26. James B. Adams, M. Baral, E. Geis, et al., "The Severity of Autism Is Associated with Toxic Metal Body Burden and Red Blood Cell Glutathione Levels," *Journal of Toxicology* 2009 (August 2009), http://www.ncbi.nlm.nih.gov/pmc/articles/PMC2809421/?tool=pubmed.

27. James B. Adams, interview with the author, October 10, 2009.

28. "Mercury Chelation to Treat Autism," National Institutes of Mental Health, last updated October 31, 2009, accessed November 25, 2011, http://clinicaltrials.gov/ct2/show/NCT00376194.

29. "Chelation Therapy Reduces Lead-Exposure Problems but Could Create Lasting Effects for Children Treated for Autism, Researchers Find," *ScienceDaily*, December 13, 2006, http://www.sciencedaily.com/releases/2006/12/061213174303.htm.

30. John Gever, "NIMH Cancels Autism Chelation Trial," *MedPage Today*, September 19, 2008, http://www.medpagetoday.com/Neurology/Autism/10979.

31. Karen Kane, "Drug Error, Not Chelation Therapy, Killed Boy, Expert Says," *Pittsburgh Post-Gazette*, January 18, 2006, http://www.post-gazette.com/pg/06018/639721.stm.

32. Duke Helfand and Alan Zarembo, "Arhem, Blue Shield to Cover Therapy for Autistic Children," Los Angeles Times, July 15, 2011, accessed January 19, 2012, http://articles.latimes.com/2011/jul/15/business/la-fi-autism-treatment-20110715.

33. James B. Adams, interview with the author, October 10, 2009.

34. Ibid.

35. "Applied Behavior Analysis (ABA)," Autism Speaks, accessed November 25, 2011, http://www.autismspeaks.org/what-autism/treatment/applied-behavior-analysis-aba.

36. "Autism Has High Cost to U.S. Society," Harvard School of Public Health, April 25, 2006, http://www.hsph.harvard.edu/news/press-releases/2006-releases/press04252006.html.

37. T. T. Shimabukuro, S. D. Grosse, and C. Rice, "Medical Expenditures for Children with an Autism Spectrum Disorder in a Privately Insured Population," Journal of Autism and Developmental Disorders 38, no. 3 (march 2008): 546–52, http://www.ncbi.nlm.nih.gov/pubmed/17690969?log$=activity.

38. Michael L. Ganz, "The Lifetime Distribution of the Incremental Societal Costs of Autism," Archives of Pediatrics and Adolescent Medicine 161, no. 4 (April 2007): 343–349, http://archpedi.ama-assn.org/cgi/content/full/161/4/343?maxtoshow=&hits=10&RESULTFORMAT=&fulltext.

39. "Parent Ratings of Behavioral Effects of Biomedical Interventions," Autism Research Institute, March 2009, http://www.autism.com/pdf/providers/ParentRatings2009.pdf.

40. "Hyperbaric oxygen therapy," Mayo Clinic, last updated October 27, 2011, accessed November 27, 2011, http://www.mayoclinic.com/health/hyperbaric-oxygen-thera-py/MY00829.
41. Marty Ann Kelley, interview with the author, October 23, 2009.
42. James B. Adams, interview with the author, October 10, 2009
43. *Refrigerator Mothers*, Film Description, PBS, last modified March 19, 2009, accessed November 25, 2011, http://www.pbs.org/pov/refrigeratormothers/film_description. php.
44. Hertz-Picciotto, "Autism & Toxic Chemical Exposure: What is the Relationship?" 2011.
45. Kristi Hogg, interview with the author, October 23, 2009.

CHAPTER FIVE: BIRTH COMPLICATIONS

1. Emma J. Glasson, Carol Bower, Beverly Petterson, Nick de Klerk, Gervase Chaney, and Joachim F. Hallmayer, "Perinatal Factors and the Development of Autism: A Population Study," *Archives of General Psychiatry* 61, no. 6 (June 2004): 618–627.
2. Emma J. Glasson, interview with the author, March 20, 2011.
3. Naya Juul-Dam, Jeanne Townsend, and Eric Courchesne, "Prenatal, Perinatal, and Neonatal Factors in Autism, Pervasive Developmental Disorder-Not Otherwise Specified, and the General Population," *Pediatrics* 107, no. 4 (April 2001): e63; http://pediatrics.aappublications.org/content/107/4/e63.full.
4. Mark Olfson and Steven C. Marcus, "National Patterns in Antidepressant Medication Treatment," *Archives of General Psychiatry* 66, no. 8 (August 2009): 848–856, http://archpsyc.ama-assn.org/cgi/content/short/66/8/848?rss=1.
5. Michael Merzenich, interview with the author, October 8, 2009.
6. Lisa A. Croen, Judith K. Grether, Cathleen K. Yoshida, Roxana Odouli, and Victoria Hendrick, "Antidepressant Use During Pregnancy and Childhood Autism Spectrum Disorders," *Archives of General Psychiatry* 68, no. 11 (November 2011): 1104–1112, http://archpsyc.ama-assn.org/cgi/content/short/archgenpsychiatry.2011.73.
7. Andrew Weeks, "Umbilical Cord Clamping After Birth," *British Medical Journal* 335, no. 7615 (August 2007): 312–313.
8. "Overview: Maternal Hemorrhage," U.S. Global Health Policy, Kaiser Family Foundation, update June 2011, accessed February 2012, http://globalhealth.kff.org/GHIR/Conditions/Maternal-Hemorrhage.aspx.
9. W. J. Prendiville, D. Elbourne, and S. McDonald, "Active Versus Expectant Management in the Third Stage of Labour," Cochrane Database od Systematic Reviews 3 (2000), 2000),http://apps.who.int/rhl/reviews/CD000007.pdf.
10. S. J. McDonald, P. Middleton, "Effect of Timing of Umbilical Cord Clamping of Term Infants on Maternal and Neonatal Outcomes," Cochrane Databaes of Systematic Reviews 2 (2008), http://apps.who.int/rhl/reviews/CD004074.pdf.
11. Judith S. Mercer, "Current Best Evidence: A Review of the Literature on Umbilical Cord Clamping," *Journal of Midwifery & Women's Health* 46, no. 6 (December 2001): 401–412, http://www.cordclamping.info/publications/LIT%20REVIEW%20AR-TICLE-MERCER.pdf.
12. Ibid.
13. Amy Romano, "Consider the Source: An interview with Cord Clamping Researcher, Judith Mercer," Science & Sensibility, November 17, 2009, http://www.scienceand-sensibility.org/?p=810.
14. Michael Merzenich, interview with the author, October 8, 2009.

15. Gemma L. Malin, Rachel K., Morris, and Khalid S. Khan, "Strength of Association Between Umbilical Cord pH and Perinatal and Long Term Outcomes: Systematic Review and Meta-Analysis," *British Medical Journal* 340 (May 2010): c1471, http://www.ncbi.nlm.nih.gov/pmc/articles/PMC2869402/.

16. Isabelle M. Rosso, Tyrone D. Cannon, Matti O. Huttunen, et al., "Obstetrics Risk Factors for Early-Onset Schizophrenia in a Finnish Birth Cohort," American Journal of Psychiatry 157 (2000): 801–807, http://ajp.psychiatryonline.org/article.aspx?Volume=157&page=801&journalID=13.

17. Dan Olmsted, "The Age of Autism: The Amish Anomaly," United Press International, http://www.whale.to/vaccine/olmsted.html.

18. Michael Merzenich, "Autism and Early Oxygen Deprivation 2," On the Brain with Dr. Mike Merzenich, PhD, June 24, 2009, http://merzenich.positscience.com/?p=248.

19. "Autism Spectrum Disorders Among Preschool Children Participating in the Minneapolis Public Schools Early Childhood Special Education Programs," Minnesota Department of Health, March 2009, http://www.health.state.mn.us/ommh/projects/autism/report090331.pdf.

20. Maura Lerner, "Autism Statistics Alarm Somalis," *Star Tribune*, last updated August 24, 2008, accessed November 26, 2011, http://www.startribune.com/lifestyle/27334979.html?source=error.

21. "Doctors Eye Vitamin D Link to Autism," UPI.com, July 15, 2008, http://www.upi.com/Science_News/2008/07/15/Doctors-eye-vitamin-D-link-to-autism/UPI-79241216154476/.

22. Merzenich, "Autism and Early Oxygen Deprivation 2," 2009.

23. Eileen K. Hutton and Eman S. Hassan, "Late vs Early Clamping of the Umbilical Cord in Full-term Neonates," *Journal of the American Medical Association* 297, no. 11 (March 2007): 1241–1252, http://www.qtnpr.ca/files/1241.pdf.

24. S. Jill James, e-mail interview with the author, April 8, 2010.

25. "Iron Deficiency's Long-Term Effects: An Interview with Pediatrician Betsy Lozoff," National Scientific Council on the Developing Child, Perspectives, 2006, http://www.pinrek.com/resources/pdf/2zl%20Iron_Deficiencys_Long_Term_Effects.pdf.

26. Richard Lathe, *Autism, Brain and Environment* (London and Philadelphia: Jessica Kingsley Publishers, 2006).

27. "Study: No Increased Autism Risk with Antenatal Ultrasound," Healthimaging, last updated September 15, 2009, accessed November 26, 2011, http://www.healthimaging.com/index.php?option=com_articles&view=article&id=18718:study-no-increased-autismrisk-with-antenatal-ultrasound.

28. R. Bowen, "Oxytocin," Colorado State University Hypertext, last updated July 12, 2010, accessed November 26, 2011, http://www.vivo.colostate.edu/hbooks/pathphys/endocrine/hypopit/oxytocin.html.

29. Tori DeAngelis, "The Two Faces of Oxytocin," *Monitor on Psychology* (American Psychology Association) 39, no. 2 (February 2008): 30, http://www.apa.org/monitor/feb08/oxytocin.aspx.

30. "HealthGrade 2011 Obstetrics & Gynecology in American Hospitals," last updated 2011, accessed January 16, 2012, http://www.healthgrades.com/business/img/HealthGrades2011ObstetricsandGynecologyinAmericanHospitalsReport.pdf.

31. Tiffany O'Callaghan, "Too Many C-Sections: Docs Rethink Induced Labor," *Time*, August 2, 2010, http://www.time.com/time/health/article/0,8599,2007754,00.html#ixzz0vSZikCgr.

32. Caroline Signore, "No Time for Complacency: Labor Inductions, Cesarean Deliveries , and the Definition of 'Term,'" Obstetrics & Gynecology 116, no. 1 (July 2010):

4–6.

33. C. Sue Carter, "Developmental Consequences of Oxytocin," *Physiology & Behavior* 79 (April 2003): 383–397, http://www.sscnet.ucla.edu/anthro/faculty/fiske/misc/carter.pdf.

34. Mary Carmichael, "The 'Bonding Hormone' That Might Cure Autism," *Newsweek*, February 25, 2010, http://www.thedailybeast.com/newsweek/2010/02/25/the-bonding-hormone-that-might-cure-autism.html.

35. David Rose and Rachel Carlyle, "Autism and Aspberger Syndrome Underdiagnosed in Women, Researchers Say," The Times (London), February 5, 2010, http://health.groups.yahoo.com/group/-AuTeach/message/3600.

36. LeeAnne Green, Deborah Fein, Charlotte Modahl, Carl Feinstein, Lynn Waterhouse, and Mariana Morris, "Oxytocin and Autistic Disorder: Alterations in Peptide Forms," *Biological Psychiatry* 50, no. 8 (2001): 609–613, http://lynnwaterhouse.intrasun.tcnj.edu/Oxytocin%20and%20Autistic%20Disorder%20alteration%20in%20peptide%20forms.pdf.

37. Eric Hollander, ed., *Autism Spectrum Disorders* (New York: Marcel Dekker, Inc., 2005).

38. Rojas Wahl and U. Roy, "Could Oxytocin Administration During Labor Contribute to Autism and Related Behavioral Disorders? A Look at the Literature," *Medical Hypotheses* 63, no. 3 (March 2004): 456–460.

39. Lisa Kurth and Robert Haussmann, "Perinatal Pitocin as an Early ADHD Biomarker: Neurodevelopmental Risk?" *Journal of Attention Disorders* 15, no. 5 (July 2011): 423–431.

40. Mike Connor, "Autism (ASD) and ADHD: Overlap and Comorbidity," The National Autistic Society, January 2008, http://www.mugsy.org/connor112.htm.

41. Ibid.

42. Simon G. Gregory, Jessica J. Connelly, Aaron J. Towers, Jessica Johnson, Dahni Biscocho, Christina A. Markuna, et al., "Genomic and Epigenetic Evidence for Oxytocin Receptor Deficiency in Autism," *BMC Medicine* 7, no. 62 (2009), http://www.biomedcentral.com/1741-7015/7/62.

43. Christopher Fisher, "Silenced Gene for Social Behavior Found in Autism that Could Serve as a Biomarker," January 13, 2010, http://www.bmedreport. com/archives/8616.

44. "Autism: Oxytocin Improves Social Behavior of Patients, Study Finds," ScienceDaily, February 16, 2010, http://www.sciencedaily.com/releases/2010/02/100216221350.htm.

45. Cindy Schultz, interview with the author, June 12, 2010.

46. Rachel Bensinger, "Hormone Could Treat Symptoms of Autism, Experts Say," *The Cornell Daily Sun*, Cornell University, February 24, 2010, http://cornellsun.com/node/41016.

47. Temple Grandin and Catherine Johnson, *Animals in Translation: Using the Mysteries of Autism to Decode Animal Behavior* (New York: Simon & Schuster, 2005).

48. M. Nagasawa, T. Kikisuim, T. Onaka, and M. Ohta, "Dog's Gaze at Its Owner Increases Owner's Urinary Oxytocin During Social Interaction," Hormones and Behavior 55, no. 3 (March 2009): 434–41, http://www.ncbi.nlm.nih.gov/pubmed/19124024.

49. François Martin and Jennifer Farnum, "Animal-Assisted Therapy for Children with Pervasive Developmental Disorders," *Western Journal of Nursing Research* 24, no. 6 (October 2002): 657–670.

50. Mona J. Sams, Elizabeth V. Fortney, and Stan Willenbring, "Occupational Therapy Incorporating Animals for Children With Autism: A Pilot Investigation," *The American Journal of Occupational Therapy* 60, no. 3 (May/June 2006): 268–274.

51. "Deadly Delivery: The Maternal Health Care Crisis in the USA," Amnesty International, 2010.
52. Ibid.
53. Carter, "Developmental Consequences of Oxytocin," 2003.

CHAPTER SIX: OUR CHEMICAL WORLD

1. Kathy Marks and Daniel Howden, "The World's Rubbish Dump: A Tip That Stretches From Hawaii to Japan," *The Independent*, February 5, 2008, http://www.independent.co.uk/environment/green-living/the-worlds-rubbishdump-a-tip-that-stretches-from-hawaii-to-japan-778016.html.
2. Michelle Allsopp, Adam Walters, David Santillo, and Paul Johnston, "Plastic Debris in the World's Oceans," Greenpeace, November 2, 2006, http://new.unep.org/regionalseas/marinelitter/publications/docs/plastic_ocean_report.pdf.
3. Malin Larsson, Bernard Weiss, Staffan Janson, Jan Sundell, and Carl-Gustav Bornehag, "Associations Between Indoor Environmental Factors and Parental-Reported Autistic Spectrum Disorders in Children 6–8 Years of Age," *Neurotoxicology* 30, no. 5 (September 2009): 822–831.
4. Bernard Weiss, interview with the author, May 12, 2010.
5. A. Miodovnik, S.M. Engel, C. Zhu, et al., "Endocrine Disruptors and Childhood Social Impairment," *Neurotoxicology* 32, no. 2 (March 2011):261–267.
6. "Review of Exposure Data and Assessments for Select Dialkyl Ortho-Phthalates," Consumer Product Safety Commission, February 24, 2010, http://www.cpsc.gov/about/cpsia/pthalexp.pdf.
7. "Phthalates Basics: Questions & Answers," American Chemistry Council, accessed November 26, 2011, http://phthalates.americanchemistry.com/Phthalates-Basics/Questions-Answers.
8. Kendra L. Howdeshell, Johnathan Furr, Christy R. Lambright, Cynthisa V. Rider, Vickie S. Wilson, and Earl Gray Jr., "Cumulative Effects of Dibutyl Phthalate on Male Rat Reproductive Tract Development: Altered Fetal Steroid Hormone and Genes," *Toxicological Sciences* 99, no. 1 (2007): 190–202, http://toxsci.oxfordjournals.org/content/99/1/190.abstract.
9. Shanna H. Swan, Katharina M. Main, Fan Liu, et al., "Decrease in Anogenital Distance among Male Infants with Prenatal Phthalate Exposure," *Environmental Health Perspectives* 113, no. 8 (August 2005): 1056–1061, http://ehp03.niehs.nih.gov/article/fetchArticle.action?articleURI=info:doi/10.1289/ehp.8100.
10. Shanna Swan, "Greening Our Children," (conference), Hyatt Regency Greenwich, May 9, 2011.
11. Ibid.
12. Dominique J. Williams, Memorandum to the US Consumer Products Safety Commission, April 7, 2010, http://www.cpsc.gov/about/cpsia/toxicityDBP.pdf.
13. Suzanne Bohan, "Phthalate Ban in Children's Products Now in Force in California," Physorg.com, January 2, 2009, http://www.physorg.com/news150097843.html.
14. "Sec. 108: Products Concerning Certain Phthalates," Consumer Product Safety Improvement Act, Consumer Products Safety Commission, December 18, 2008, http://www.cpsc.gov/about/cpsia/faq/108faq.html.
15. "Public Health Statement for Polychlorinated Biphenyls (PCBs)," Agency for Toxic Substances & Disease Registry, November 2000, http://www.atsdr.cdc.gov/phs/phs.asp?id=139&tid=26.
16. "Hudson River Natural Resource Damage Assessment Plan," Hudson River Trustee

Council, September 2002, http://www.fws.gov/contaminants/restorationplans/ hudsonriver/docs/HudsonRiverNRDASept2002.pdf.

17. Nicoletta Borghesi, Simonetta Corsolini, and Silvano Focardi, "Levels of Polybrominated Diphenyl Ethers (PBDEs) and Polychlorinated Biphenyls (PCBs) in Two Species of Antarctic Fish (*Chionodraco hamatus* and *Trematomus bernacchii*)," Department of Environmental Science (University of Siena), 2007, http://www.bfr2010. com/abstract-download/2007/P035.pdf.

18. Jennifer O'Brien, "Class of PCBs Causes Developmental Abnormalities in Rat Pups," University of California, San Francisco, April 23, 2007, http://www.ucsf.edu/ news/2007/04/5564/class-pcbs-causes-developmental-abnormalities-rat-pups.

19. Merzenich, interview with the author, 2009.

20. Jeff Miller, "Breastfeeding, Brain Development and Chemical Poisons: Neuroscientist Michael Merzenich," University of California, San Francisco, May 18, 2007, http:// www.ucsf.edu/news/2007/05/3817/merzenich.

21. Margaret M. McDowell, Chia-Yih Wang, and Jocelyn Kennedy-Stephenson, "Breastfeedingin the United States: Findings from the National Health and Nu- trition Examination Survey, 1999–2006," NCHS Data Brief no. 5, Centers for Disease Control and Prevention, April 2008, http://www.cdc.gov/nchs/data/databriefs/db05.htm.

22. J. S. Woods, M. D. Martin, C. A. Naleway, and D. Echeverria, "Urinary Porphyrin Profiles as a Biomarker of Mercury Exposure: Studies on Dentists with Occupational Exposure to Mercury Vapor," Journal of Toxicology and Environmental Health 40. No. 2-3 (October 1993): 235–46, http://www.ncbi.nlm.nih.gov/pubmed/8230299.

23. James S.Woods, Sarah E. Armel, Denise I. Fulton, et al., "Urinary Porphyrin Excretion in Neurotypical and Autistic Children," *Environmental Health Perspectives* 118, no. 10 (October 2010): 1450–1457, http://ehp03.niehs.nih.gov/article/fetchArticle.action?a rticleURI=info%3Adoi%2F10.1289%2Fehp.0901713.

24. J. K. Kern, D. A. Geier, J. B. Adams, M. R. Geier, "A Biomarker of Mercury Body-Burden Correlated with Diagnostic Domain Specific Clinical Symptoms of Autism Spectrum Disorder," Biometals 23, no. 6 (December 2010): 1043-51, http://www.ncbi. nlm.nih.gov/pubmed/20532957.

25. "A Survey of Bisphenol A in US Canned Foods," Environmental Working Group, March 5, 2007, http://www.ewg.org/reports/bisphenola.

26. "Concern Over Canned Foods," *Consumer Reports Magazine*, December 2009, http://www.consumerreports.org/cro/magazine-archive/december-2009/food/ bpa/overview/bisphenol-a-ov.htm.

27. "Fact Sheet: Bisphenol A (BPA)," Centers for Disease Control and Prevention, last updated February 28, 2011, accessed November 26, 2011, http://www.cdc.gov/exposurereport/BisphenolA_FactSheet.html.

28. Kellyn S. Betts, "Body of Proof: Biomonitoring Data Reveal Widespread Bisphenol A Exposures," Environmental Health Perspectives 118, no. 8 (August 2010): A353, http://www.ncbi.nlm.nih.gov/pmc/articles/PMC2920109/.

29. "Bisphenol A (BPA) Action Plan Summary," US Environmental Protection Agency, last updated September 12, 2011, accessed November 26, 2011, http://www.epa.gov/ opptintr/existingchemicals/pubs/actionplans/bpa.html.

30. "History of Bisphenol A," University of Minnesota, last modified December 15, 2008, accessed November 26, 2011, http://enhs.umn.edu/current/2008studentwebsites/ pubh6101/bpa/history.html.

31. Doug Hamilton, "Interview: Frederick Vom Saal, PhD," Frontline, February 1998, http://www.pbs.org/wgbh/pages/frontline/shows/nature/interviews/vomsaal.html.

32. Richard W. Stahlhut, Wade V. Welshons, and Shanna S. Swan, "Bisphenol A Data

in NHANES Suggest Longer than Expected Half-Life, Substantial Nonfood Exposure, or Both," *Environmental Health Perspectives* 117, no. 5 (May 2009), http://ehp03. niehs.nih.gov/article/fetchArticle.action?articleURI=info:doi/10.1289/ehp.080037.

33. Sonya Lunder, David Andrews, and Jane Houlihan, "Synthetic Estrogen BPA Coats Cash Register Receipts," Environmental Working Group, July 27, 2010, http://www. ewg.org/bpa-in-store-receipts.

34. "NTP-CERHR Monograph on the Potential Human and Reproductive Developmental Effects of Bisphenol A," Center for the Evaluation of Risks to Human Reproduction, National Toxicology Program, September 2008, http://ntp.niehs.nih.gov/ ntp/ohat/bisphenol/bisphenol.pdf.

35. BATTF (Bisphenol A Toxicology Task Force), "Bisphenol A: Summary of the Key Toxicology Studies, Estrogenicity Data and an Evaluation of the No-Observed-Effect-Level (NOEL)," The Society of the Plastics Industry, Inc., Washington, D.C., February 9, 1995.

36. "Update on Bisphenol A for Use in Food Contact Applications: January 2010," US Food and Drug Administration, last updated March 22, 2010, accessed November 26, 2011, http:// www.fda.gov/NewsEvents/PublicHealthFocus/ucm197739.htm#current.

37. Elizabeth Kolbert, "A Warning by Key Researcher on Risks of BPA in Our Lives," *Yale Environment* 360, November 24, 2010, http://e360.yale.edu/feature/a_warning_by_ key_researcher_on_risks_of_bpa_in_our_lives/2344/.

38. A. Miodovnik, S. M. Engel, C. Zhu, et al., "Endocrine Disruptors and Childhood Social Impairment," *Neurotoxicology* 32, no. 2 (March 2011): 261–267, http://www. ncbi.nlm.nih.gov/pubmed/21182865.

39. Ibid.

40. Ibid.

41. "Epigenetics," NOVA, July 1, 2007, http://www.pbs.org/wgbh/nova/body/epigenetics.html.

42. Jill U. Adams, "Obesity, Epigenetics and Gene Regulation," *Nature Education* 1, no. 1 (2008), http://www.nature.com/scitable/topicpage/obesity-epigenetics-andgene-regulation-927.

43. Shuk-mei Ho, interview with the author, May 2010.

44. "Human Epigenome Project," Human Epigenome Project, accessed November 26 2011, http://www.epigenome.org/index.php?page=project.

45. S. Jill James, Stepan Melnyk, Stefanie Jernigan, et al., "Abnormal Transmethylation/ Transsulfuration Metabolism and DNA Hypomethylation Among Parents of Children with Autism," *Journal of Autism and Developmental Disorders* 38, no. 10 (November 2008): 1966–1975, http://www.ncbi.nlm.nih.gov/pmc/articles/PMC2584168/.

46. Laura S. Schultz, "The Dutch Hunger Winter and the Developmental Origins of Health and Disease," Proceedings of the National Academy of Sciences of the United States of America 107, no. 39 (September 28, 2010): 16757–16758, http://www.pnas. org/content/107/39/16757.full.

47. Martina Barnevik–Olsson, Christopher Gillberg, and Elisabeth Fernell, "Prevalence of Autism in Children Born to Somali Parents Living in Sweden: A Brief Report," *Developmental Medicine & Child Neurology* 50, no. 8 (August 2008): 598–601, http:// onlinelibrary.wiley.com/doi/10.1111/j.1469-8749.2008.03036.x/pdf.

48. "Autism and the Somali Community—Report of Study Fact Sheet," Minnesota Department of Health, accessed January 12, 2012, http://www.health.state.mn.us/ ommh/projects/autism/reportfs090331.cfm.

49. Matthew D. Anway, Charles Leathers, and Michael K. Skinner, "Endocrine Disruptor Vinclozolin Induced Epigenetic Transgenerational Adult-Onset Disease," *En-*

docrinology 147, no. 12 (December 2006): 5515, http://endo.endojournals.org/content/147/12/5515.full.

50. "R.E.D. Facts: Vinclozolin," US Environmental Protection Agency, October 2000, http://www.epa.gov/oppsrrd1/REDs/factsheets/2740fact.pdf.

51. Ibid.

52. "Dichlorodiphenyltrichloroethane," Report on Carcinogens, Twelfth Edition (2011), http://ntp.niehs.nih.gov/ntp/roc/twelfth/profiles/Dichlorodiphenyltrichloroethane.pdf.

53. Rachel Carson, *Silent Spring* (New York: First Mariner Books, 1962).

54. Jack Lewis, "The Birth of EPA," US Environmental Protection Agency, November 1985, http://www.epa.gov/aboutepa/history/topics/epa/15c.html.

55. "DDT Ban Takes Effect," press release, US Environmental Protection Agency, December 31, 1972, http://www.rst2.edu/ties/DDTS/university/docs/epa1.pdf.

56. "ToxFAQs for DDT, DDE, and DDD," 2002.

57. Eric M. Roberts, Paul B. English, Judith K. Grether, et al., "Maternal Residence Near Agricultural Pesticide Applications and Autism Spectrum Disorders among Children in the California Central Valley," *Environmental Health Perspectives* 115, no. 10 (October 2007), http://ehp03.niehs.nih.gov/article/fetchArticle.action?articleURI=info:doi/10.1289/ehp.10168.

58. Julie Karceski, "A California Cluster," E – The Environmental Magazine, Jan./Feb. 2012, http://www.emagazine.com/magazine-archive/a-california-cluster.

59. "Geneticists Find Location of Major Gene in ADHD; Also Linked to Autism," ScienceBlog, October 22, 2002, http://scienceblog.com/205/geneticists-findlocation-of-major-gene-in-adhd-also-linked-to-autism/.

60. Amy Marks, Kim Harley, Asa Bradman, Katherine Kogut, Dana Boyd Barr, et al., "Organophosphate Pesticide Exposure and Attention in Young Mexican-American Children: The CHAMACOS Study," Environmental Health Perspectives 118, no. 12 (December 2010), http://ehsehplp03.niehs.nih.gov/article/fetchArticle.action?articl eURI=info%3Adoi%2F10.1289%2Fehp.1002056.

61. Ibid.

62. Caroline Helwick, "More Evidence Organophosphate Pesticides Raise ADHD Risk in Children," MedScape, August 20, 2010, http://www.medscape.com/viewarticle/727225.

63. Marlene Busko, "Antiflea Pet Shampoos with Pyrethrin May Play a Role in Autism," Medscape, May 20, 2008, http://www.medscape.com/viewarticle/574799.

64. "Pyrethrins and Pyrethroids," National Pesticide Telecommunications Network, December 1998, http://npic.orst.edu/factsheets/pyrethrins.pdf.

65. Virginia A. Rauh, Robin Garfinkel, Frederica P. Perera, et al., "Impact of Prenatal Chlorpyrifos Exposure on Neurodevelopment in the First 3 Years of Life Among Inner-City Children," *Pediatrics* 118, no. 6 (December 2006): e1845–e1859, http://www.ipminstitute.org/Fed_Agency_Resources/rauh_chlorpyrifos_pediatrics.pdf.

66. Ibid.

67. Ibid.

68. "Reducing Pesticide Exposure in Children and Pregnant Women," *Northwest Bulletin* 21, no. 1 (Fall/Winter 2006): 1–15, http://depts.washington.edu/nwbfch/PDFs/NWBv21n1.pdf.

69. "Chlorpyrifos Facts," US Environmental Protection Agency, February 2002, http://www.epa.gov/pesticides/reregistration/REDs/factsheets/chlorpyrifos_fs.htm.

70. Helwick, "More Evidence Organophosphate Pesticides Raise ADHD Risk in Children," 2010.

71. "An Open Letter to President Barack Obama," Rachel Carson Council, March 25, 2009, http://www.rachelcarsoncouncil.org/uploads/articles/RCC%20Open%20Letter%20to%20Obama.pdf.

72. Susanne Rust, "Connecticut Bans BPA," *Journal Sentinel*, June 4, 2009, http://www.jsonline.com/blogs/news/47001387.html.

73. "Consumers Union & Environmental Working Group Commend CA Senate Health Committee for Passing BPA Ban; Urge Swift Passage by Senate," ConsumersUnion, last updated June 22, 2011, accessed January 16, 2012, http://www.consumersunion.org/pub/core_food_safety/017830.html.

74. "California BPA Ban Signed Into Law," Food Safety News, October 6, 2011, http://www.foodsafetynews.com/2011/10/california-bpa-ban-signed-by-gov-brown/.

75. "Conn. Bans Receipts Containing BPA," Plast-world.com, June 11, 2011, http://www.plast-world.com/conn-bans-receipts-containing-bpa-2827-news

76. Lyndsey Layton, "No BPA for Baby Bottles in US," *The Washington Post*, March 6, 2009, http://www.washingtonpost.com/wp-dyn/content/article/2009/03/05/AR2009030503285.html.

77. Susanne Rust and Meg Kissinger, "Maker Acknowledges BPA Worries," *Journal Sentinel*, March 12, 2009, http://www.jsonline.com/watchdog/watchdogreports/41186522.html.

78. Sen. Dianne Feinstein, "Chemical Industry Lobbyists Block Measure to Protect Infants and Toddlers," *The Huffington Post*, November 19, 2010, http://www.huffingtonpost.com/sen-dianne-feinstein/chemical-industry-lobbyis_b_785930.html.

79. "Toxic Substances Control Act," US Code online via GPO Access, last updated December 23, 2008, accessed November 26, 2011, http://frwebgate.access.gpo.gov/cgi-bin/usc.cgi?ACTION=RETRIEVE&FILE=$$xa$$busc15.wais&start=9588738&SIZE=4446&TYPE=TEXT.

80. "US Chemical Management: The Toxic Substances Control Act," Physicians for Social Responsibility, accessed November 26, 2011, http://www.psr.org/environment-and-health/confronting-toxics/chemical-management/.

81. Swan, "Greening Our Children," 2011.

82. Sheila Kaplan, "Reform of Toxic Chemicals Law Collapses as Industry Flexes Its Muscles," *Politics Daily*, October 13, 2010, http://www.politicsdaily.com/2010/10/13/reform-of-toxic-chemicals-law-collapses-as-industry-flexes-its-m/

83. Ibid.

84. "Bisphenol A: Toxic Plastics Chemical in Canned Food: Companies Reduced BPA Exposures in Japan," Environmental Working Group, accessed November 26, 2011, http://www.ewg.org/node/20938.

85. "REACH," European Commission Environment, last updated November 16, 2011, accessed November 26, 2011, http://ec.europa.eu/environment/chemicals/reach/reach_intro.htm.

86. "Six Chemicals in Soft Plastic Toys Banned Across Europe," *Environment News Service*, July 6, 2005, http://www.ens-newswire.com/ens/jul2005/2005-07-06-05.html.

87. Jayne O'Donnell, "Furniture to be Greener, but Pricier," *USA Today*, March 13, 2011, http://www.usatoday.com/printedition/money/20100719/formaldehyde19_st.art.htm.

88. Marla Cone, "US Rules Allow the Sale of Products Others Ban," *Los Angeles Times*, October 8, 2006, http://www.commondreams.org/headlines06/1008-01.htm.

89. Noelle Robbins, "Not a Pretty Picture," *Earth Island Journal*, Spring 2011, accessed November 26, 2011, http://eii.org/journal/index.php/eij/article/not_a_pretty_picture/.

90. "Are Pharmaceuticals in Your Watershed? Understanding the Fate of Pharmaceuticals and Other Contaminants in Watersheds," US Geological Survey, last modified November 12, 2010, accessed November 26, 2011, http://toxics.usgs.gov/highlights/pharm_watershed/.
91. Ibid.
92. "Triclosan Fact Sheet," Congressman Ed Markey, accessed November 26, 2011, http://markey.house.gov/docs/triclosan_information_final.pdf.
93. "Commission Decision," Official Journal of the European Union, March 3, 2010, accessed February 3, 2012, http://eur-lex.europa.eu/LexUriServ/LexUriServ.do?uri=O J:L:2010:075:0025:0026:EN:PDF.
94. "Triclosan Fact Sheet," Congressman Ed Markey, 2011.
95. "April 13, 2010: Markey Urges Major Companies to Remove Triclosan from Consumer Soaps, Other Products," Congressman Ed Markey, accessed November 26, 2011, http://markey.house.gov/index.php?option=content&task=view&id=3965&Item id=125.
96. Lisa Huguenin, "Autism & Toxic Chemical Exposure: What is the Relationship?" (teleconference), Safer Chemicals Healthy Families, June 7, 2011.
97. Angel Jennings, "Thomas the Tank Engine Toys Recalled Because of Lead Paint," The New York Times, June 15, 2007, http://www.nytimes.com/2007/06/15/business/15recall.html.
98. David Schaper, "Thomas the Tank Engine Recall Angers Parents," NPR, June 22, 2007, http://www.npr.org/templates/story/story.php?storyId=11271805.
99. "Spin Master Recalls Aqua Dots—Children Became Unconscious After Swallowing Beads," US Consumer Product Safety Commission, November 7, 2007, http://www.cpsc.gov/cpscpub/prerel/prhtml08/08074.html.
100. Huguenin, "Autism & Toxic Chemical Exposure: What is the Relationship?" 2011.

CHAPTER SEVEN: UNANSWERED QUESTIONS

1. Douglas Fischer, Kim Hooper, Maria Athanasiadou, Ioannis Athanassiadis, and Ake Bergman, "Children Show Highest Levels of Polybrominated Diphenyl Ethers in a California Family of Four: A Case Study," Environmental Health Perspectives 114, no. 10 (October 2006): 1581–1584, http://ehp03.niehs.nih.gov/article/fetchArticle.actio n?articleURI=info%3Adoi%2F10.1289%2Fehp.8554.
2. "Public Health Statement for Polybrominated Diphenyl Ethers (PBDEs)," Agency for Toxic Substances & Disease Registry, September 2004, http://www.atsdr.cdc.gov/phs/phs.asp?id=899&tid=94.
3. Douglas Fischer, "It's In Us All," Oakland Tribune, March 27, 2006, http://www.insidebayarea.com/oaklandtribune/localnews/ci_3299744.
4. Merzenich, interview with the author, 2009.
5. "Public Health Statement for Polybrominated Diphenyl Ethers (PBDEs)," 2004.
6. Patricia O'Campo, interview with the author, 2010.
7. Pam Belluck, "Wanted: Volunteers, All Pregnant," The New York Times, February 15, 2010, http://www.nytimes.com/2010/02/16/health/16child.html.
8. "What Is the National Children's Study?" The National Children's Study, last updated November 3, 2011, accessed November 26, 2011, http://www.nationalchildrensstudy.gov/about/overview/Pages/default.aspx.
9. Philip J. Landrigan, "Greening Our Children" (conference), slideshow, May 9, 2011, http://www.mountsinai.org/static_files/MSMC/Files/Patient%20Care/Children/Childrens%20Environmental%20Health%20Center/Landrigan%20GoC_

slides%20Sunday%20PM.pdf.

10. "What You Need to Know about Mercury in Fish and Shellfish," US Environmental Protection Agency, 2004, http://water.epa.gov/scitech/swguidance/fishshellfish/outreach/advice_index.cfm.

11. "Frequently Asked Questions About Produce and Pesticides," Environmental Working Group, accessed November 26, 2011, http://www.ewg.org/foodnews/faq/.

12. "EWG's 2011 Shopper's Guide to Pesticides in Produce," Environmental Working Group, accessed November 26, 2011, http://www.ewg.org/foodnews/.

13. "Draft Risk Assessment of the Potential Human Health Effects Associated with Exposure to Perfluorooctanoic Acid and Its Salts," U.S. Environmental Protection Agency Office of Pollution Prevention and Toxics Risk Assessment Division," January 4, 2005, http://www.epa.gov/oppt/pfoa/pubs/pfoarisk.pdf.

14. Benjamin J. Apelberg, Frank R. Witter, Julie B. Herbstman, Antonia M. Calafat, Rolf U. Halden, Larry L. Needham, and Lynn R. Goldman, "Cold Serum Concentrations of Perfluorooctane Sulfonate (PFOS) and Perfluorooctanoate (PFOA) in Relation to Weight and Size at Birth," Environmental Health Perspectives 115, no. 11 (November 2007), http://ehp03.niehs.nih.gov/article/info:doi/10.1289/ehp.10334.

15. "Perfluorooctanoic Acid (PFOA) and Fluorinated Telomers," US Environmental Protection Agency, last updated September 22, 2011, accessed November 26, 2011, http://www.epa.gov/oppt/pfoa/pubs/pfoainfo.html#actions.

16. David Lazarus, "Worries Stick to Food Packing," Los Angeles Times, July 30, 2008, http://articles.latimes.com/2008/jul/30/business/fi-lazarus30.

17. "Chemical Cuisine: Learn About Food Additives," Center for Science in the Public Interest, accessed November 26, 2011, http://www.cspinet.org/reports/chemcuisine.htm.

18. Sheela Sathyanarayana, Catherine J. Karr, Paula Lozano, et al., "Baby Care Products: Possible Sources of Infant Phthalate Exposure," Pediatrics 121, no. 2 (February 2008): e260–e268, http://pediatrics.aappublications.org/content/121/2/e260.full?maxtosho w=&hits=10&RESULTFORMAT=&fulltext=phthalates&searchid=1&FIRSTIND EX=0&sortspec=relevance&resourcetype=HWCIT.

19. Ruthann A. Rudel, Janet M. Gray, Connie L. Engel, et al., "Food Packaging and Bisphenol A and Bis(2-Ethyhexyl) Phthalate Exposure: Findings from a Dietary Intervention," Environmental Health Perspectives 119, no. 7 (July 2011): 914–920, http://ehp03.niehs.nih.gov/article/info:doi/10.1289/ehp.1003170.

20. "How to Reduce BPA Levels by 60 Percent in 3 Days," Safer Chemicals Healthy Families Blog, March 31, 2011, http://blog.saferchemicals.org/2011/03/how-to-reduce-bpa-levels-by-60-percent-in-3-days.html.

21. "Lead in Lipstick," Campaign for Safe Cosmetics, accessed November 27, 2011, http://safecosmetics.org/article.php?id=223.

22. "Lipstick and Lead: Questions and Answers," US Food and Drug Administration, last updated November 3, 2009, accessed November 26, 2011, http://www.fda.gov/Cosmetics/ProductandIngredientSafety/ProductInformation/ucm137224.htm.

23. David C. Bellinger, "Very Low Lead Exposures and Children's Neurodevelopment," Pediatrics 20, no. 2 (April 2008): 172–177.

24. "Beauty Industry Lobbies to Keep Lead in Lipstick," The Campaign for Safe Cosmetics, June 26, 2008, http://www.safecosmetics.org/article.php?id=249.

25. "EWG's Skin Deep Database," Environmental Working Group, accessed November 25, 2011, http://www.ewg.org/skindeep/.

26. "Trihalomethanes in Drinking Water," Government of Quebec, Canada, 2009, accessed November 26, 2011, http://publications.msss.gouv.qc.ca/acrobat/f/

documentation/2009/09-239-01A.pdf.

27. Mireya Navarro, "Higher Levels of Lead Seen in City Tap Water," The New York Times, November 4, 2010, http://www.nytimes.com/2010/11/05/nyregion/05lead.html.

28. "Run Your Tap," poster, NYC Department of Environmental Protection, 2011, http://www.nyc.gov/html/dep/pdf/lead/dep_run_your_tap_poster.pdf.

29. "What's on Tap?" Natural Resources Defense Council, accessed November 26, 2011, http://www.nrdc.org/water/drinking/uscities/execsum.asp.

30. Rita Savard, "'Natural' Doesn't Always Mean 'Safe,'" Lowell Sun, March 6, 2006, http://www.uml.edu/News/news-articles/2006/natural_doesnt_al.aspx.

31. "Reducing Pesticide Exposure in Children and Pregnant Women," 2006.

32. Mae Wu, Mayra Quirindongo, Jennifer Sass, and Andrew Wetzler, "Still Poisoning the Well," Natural Resources Defense Council, April 2010, http://www.nrdc.org/health/atrazine/files/atrazine10.pdf.

33. "Keeping Our Waters Safe: The 112th Congress Must Not Strip the EPA's Duty to Protect Our Waters from Pesticides," Natural Resources Defense Council, last modified March 23, 2011, accessed November 26, 2011, http://www.nrdc.org/legislation/keepingourwatersafe.asp.

34. "Safe Cosmetics Act of 2011 Introduced in Congress," Safer Chemicals Healthy Families Blog, June 28, 2011, http://blog.saferchemicals.org/2011/06/safe-cosmetics-act-of-2011-introduced-in-congress.html.

35. Andy Igrejas, interview with the author, July 8, 2011.

INDEX

❖

•

ABOUT THE AUTHOR

❖

Brita Belli is the editor of *E – The Environmental Magazine*, an independent magazine dedicated to green issues. Prior to joining *E*, Brita was the arts editor at the *Fairfield County Weekly*, where she won numerous awards for her writing. She wrote the book *The Complete Idiot's Guide to Renewable Energy for Your Home*, and her stories have been featured in the books *Notes from the Underground: The Most Outrageous Stories from the Alternative Press* and *Best AltWeekly Writing and Design 2006*; she also edited the book *EarthTalk: Expert Answers to Everyday Questions About the Environment*. Brita has written columns on green issues for the *Union of Concerned Scientists* and *Connecticut Home & Garden*, and her articles have appeared in *Plenty Magazine*, MSN.com, Treehugger.com, *Fairfield Magazine*, *Colorado Springs Independent*, *Black & White City Paper*, *Illinois Times*, and *Monterey County Weekly*. She has appeared on numerous TV programs as an eco-expert, and maintains a blog on autism and the environment at www.autismandtoxins.com.

ABOUT SEVEN STORIES PRESS

❖

Seven Stories Press is an independent book publisher based in New York City. We publish works of the imagination by such writers as Nelson Algren, Russell Banks, Octavia E. Butler, Ani DiFranco, Assia Djebar, Ariel Dorfman, Coco Fusco, Barry Gifford, Hwang Sok-yong, Lee Stringer, and Kurt Vonnegut, to name a few, together with political titles by voices of conscience, including the Boston Women's Health Collective, Noam Chomsky, Angela Y. Davis, Human Rights Watch, Derrick Jensen, Ralph Nader, Loretta Napoleoni, Gary Null, Project Censored, Barbara Seaman, Alice Walker, Gary Webb, and Howard Zinn, among many others. Seven Stories Press believes publishers have a special responsibility to defend free speech and human rights, and to celebrate the gifts of the human imagination, wherever we can. For additional information, visit www.sevenstories.com.